White Coats

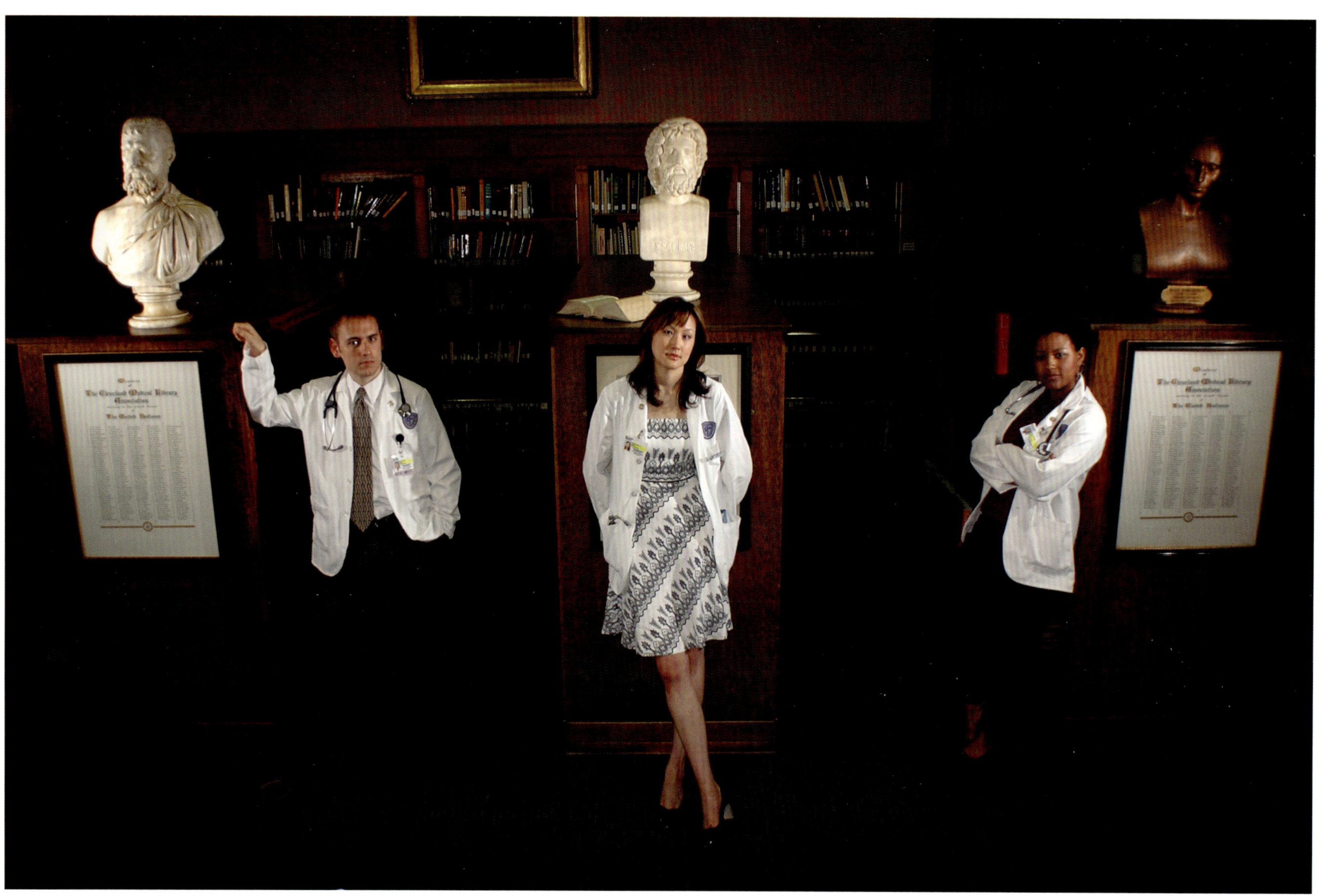

White Coats

Three Journeys through an American Medical School

Jacqueline Marino

Photographs by Tim Harrison

The Kent State University Press ⊠ Kent, Ohio

For Stella and Charlotte

Frontis: Michael Norton, Millie Gentry, and Marleny Franco, students from the Case Western Reserve University School of Medicine's class of 2009. They were photographed at the Allen Memorial Library on June 27, 2006.

Library of Congress Catalog Card Number 2011047799
ISBN 978-1-60635-130-7
Manufactured in China

The material in this book was originally published in a substantially different form in the August and September 2006, August 2007, August 2008, and August 2009 issues of *Cleveland Magazine* as a feature series entitled "White Coats." Permission from *Cleveland Magazine* is gratefully acknowledged.

LIBRARY OF CONGRESS CATALOGING-IN-PUBLICATION DATA
Marino, Jacqueline.
White coats : three journeys through an American medical school / Jacqueline Marino ; photographs by Tim Harrison.
p. cm.
ISBN 978-1-60635-130-7 (hardcover : alk. paper) ∞
1. Medical students—Ohio—Case studies. 2. Medical education—Ohio. 3. Medical colleges—Ohio. 4. Case Western Reserve University. School of Medicine. I. Title.
R747.C292M37 2012
610.71'1771—dc23 2011047799

16 15 14 13 12 5 4 3 2 1

Honor the physician with the honor due him,
according to your need of him,
for the Lord created him;
for healing comes from the Most High,
and he will receive a gift from the king.
The skill of the physician lifts up his head,
and in the presence of great men he is admired.

—Ecclesiasticus 38:1–3

There is no magic moment in which the student, as an understudy to a great actor who falls ill, is thrust on to the stage. Modern medicine is too well organized for that. The transition, from young layman aspiring to be a physician to the young physician skilled in technique and sure of his part in dealing with patients in the complex setting of modern clinics and hospitals, is slow and halting. The young man finds out quite soon that he must learn first to be a medical student; how he will act in the future, when he is a doctor, is not his immediate problem.

—Becker, Geer, Hughes, and Strauss,
Boys in White: Student Culture in Medical School

Contents

Author's Note

We call on physicians at birth and death and every significant medical event in between, but we rarely consider the personal challenges faced by those on their way to becoming our sages and saviors. From 2005 through 2009, I followed three students as they became doctors at the Case Western Reserve University School of Medicine. The resulting series, "White Coats," appeared in *Cleveland Magazine* in five separate issues over four years.

From the beginning, I focused on the human challenges involved in becoming a doctor. Regardless of curriculum or culture, a transformation takes place. I brought the readers into the settings of this transformation—the anatomy labs, classrooms, and hospitals where the students beheld their first cadavers, took their first pulses, and witnessed their first births. I explained significant issues in medical education through the students' struggles to master the ever-increasing load of medical science, confront problems of professionalism, and learn the importance of empathy. I also chronicled the students' personal sacrifices—crushing debt, round-the-clock work, and neglect of family, friends, and health. The series revolved around one question: "How does one grow into the white coat?"

In this book, I revisit the reporting I did over four years and add more history and context, as well as details that didn't make the magazine series, which was limited by space restraints. As a result, the book includes more research and greater insights.

Like anyone reading this, I have turned to doctors in times of need. I have been a patient and a family member of patients, and I will be again. The way doctors are educated affects us all. I reported on medical school from the medical students' perspectives, but I also told their stories as factually as possible. I approached this project as a reporter, double-checking the things students told me and running them through the why-anyone-else-should-care filter.

The audience for this book is medical educators and those considering medical school. But it is also a book for those who wonder about the personal challenges confronting the future doctors who will one day treat their cancer, alleviate their pain, and put them back together after car crashes. This work can help patients better understand their doctors. With understanding comes empathy, and—I hope—better doctor-patient relationships.

We are at a time, once again, of change in both medical school and health care in general. No matter what happens with legislation governing medical practice, however, doctors must continue to meet society's expectations of them. The specifics of how they are trained will evolve—the process by which my three subjects were educated just a few years ago has already changed—but those societal expectations will remain high, as they should for those society trusts with scalpels and prescription privileges. The book describes scenes that I observed and others that were reconstructed according to the students' own memories and writings. When possible, I also interviewed patients, doctors, faculty, family members, friends, and others who were also present. All three of the students reviewed their parts of the book for accuracy before it was published.

The result is not a complete history of these students' four years in medical school. Only full immersion in their lives would have made me qualified to produce such a work. Instead, I relay experiences that affected the students in ways significant to their development as physicians. Many of these experiences revolve around certain key themes other authors have noted in works about medical school, such as the immense quantity of material that must be learned, the intimate confrontation with death, and the indoctrination into the culture of medicine.

What goes into earning the long white coat is changing, but growing into it remains an astonishing feat. This work proves it.

Prologue

Doctors used to wear black. Like priests, they were called when sick people were out of other options. In the mid-nineteenth century, doctors still opened veins with spring-loaded lancets and bled arms over the indented lips of white basins. They still blistered and scarred. Before they knew how to prevent infection in surgery, they still operated with unsterilized knives and bone saws, their handles made of ivory, ebony, and tortoise shell. These tools arrived from London and Paris in special surgical kits, some made of mahogany and lined with velvet. The tools, like the kits, were beautiful, but as dangerous as the hands that wielded them.

At that time, getting a medical education was not difficult. Medical schools operated for profit, sometimes above a corner drugstore. Instruction was not rigorous. There were no entrance exams, no grades. Students were made doctors after listening to lectures, reading textbooks, and doing whatever clinical duties their doctor-instructors (called preceptors) required—mixing herbs, bandaging wounds, physically restraining patients during operations.

In Ohio, preceptors did not require human dissection. It was illegal until 1881. Before then, if students or instructors wanted to dissect a body, they had to steal one (or have one stolen) from a graveyard, and some did, adding "grave robber" to the other unflattering descriptions of doctors in the nineteenth century. In general, doctors did not take on the air of respectability they hold today until the late 1800s, around the same time they started wearing the long white coat.

More than the stethoscope and the serpent on the staff, the white coat remains the leading symbol of the doctor. Every student at the Case Western Reserve University School of Medicine receives one. The short white coat falls just past the hips. It is 65 percent polyester, 35 percent cotton, and machine washable only if the student doesn't care how it looks in four years. It collects makeup, dirt, and more germs than anyone wants to know. It makes students feel both big and small—big because outside the medical profession, the few inches of fabric that distinguish medical students from degreed doctors don't matter much, small because inside the medical profession, the short coat signals they are students. No one expects them to know what they're doing yet, them least of all.

Each summer, new medical students receive their coats at the White Coat Ceremony, which at Case dates back only to 1996. It takes place at Severance Hall, home of the Cleveland Orchestra and the most elegant venue in the city. It is, according to the *New Yorker* writer Charles Michener, "the most intimate of America's great symphony halls. The walls have no right angles, and the stage bellies out, as if to lock the audience in an embrace." On that affectionate stage, physicians in long white coats help the students into their short white ones. Teachers do not dress their students in any other profession. In medicine, however, it makes sense. Doctors must touch their patients. They cut open their flesh, manipulate their organs, and count the components of their blood. The good ones don't just see patients; they treat them. "Treat" is a word signaling compassion, and touch is its best sense. At the symbolic start to medical school, the physical interaction between teacher and student cements the relationship on which modern medical education is based. The knowledge of the older generation must be passed down in ways both formal and informal. The simple act of helping with the coat—the slipping of arms into sleeves, the tugging of fabric over shoulders—shows students they are not alone in acts significant and insignificant. These older doctors will teach them not just to heal but to touch.

After that first time in front of their teachers, colleagues, family, and friends, the students will put on the coat themselves, privately, for the most part. The garment will assume whatever power patients give it. The students can only try to measure up.

The Students

One April afternoon in 2005, I made a bold request to the deans of Cleveland's Case Western Reserve University School of Medicine. We were sitting around a large conference table in the Richard F. Celeste Biomedical Research Building, a red-brick clock tower set far back from the unyielding traffic of Adelbert Road. An associate editor at *Cleveland Magazine* at the time, I was joined at the table by Dean Ralph Horwitz, several other deans, and the sympathetic public affairs director, who had managed weeks of back-and-forth e-mails among us all. Horwitz wore a pair of glasses that kept distracting me—the frames looked splashed with brightly colored paint. I quietly shredded my cuticles under the table.

I want unlimited access to every classroom, lab, and clinical setting where first-year students learn medicine, I finally said. I want to show what it takes for someone to make it through the first year of medical school.

I presented my project as an opportunity for an honest look at the first year through the eyes of several first-year students. The deans seemed intrigued but a little thrown when I said I wanted to shadow their students for an entire year, and I would not permit anyone from the school to review what I would publish.

The deans kept lobbing question after question—the way they might if I were competing for one of their highly coveted short white coats. Horwitz and the other deans wanted to know why I wished to write this story. I didn't have an "elevator pitch" reason. I told them that I have several family members in the medical profession, and I'd always been intrigued by their stories. But I couldn't call myself a card-carrying medical writer. I graduated from journalism school in 1994 and spent a year in San Francisco working as an AmeriCorps VISTA volunteer at a nonprofit arts center. I started my professional journalism career in 1996 working at alternative weekly newspapers, where I had to learn to write fast and long about everything.

I didn't tell them this, but the late Dennis Freeland, my editor at the *Memphis Flyer*, where I worked from 1996 to 1999, used to tease me about being the paper's "conscience" because I often chose to write about perceived injustices and societal outcasts, including the mentally ill and inmates in the overcrowded county jail. Dennis always published those stories, though, and in 1998, not long after the Bosnian War ended, he encouraged me to report on a medical mission to Belgrade for the *Flyer*'s sister publication, *Memphis Magazine.* Many journalists recall a formative experience early in their careers, the one that reaffirms their decision not to go to law school. The Belgrade assignment was mine. Trying not to trip over the hem of my oversized scrubs (the only ones available) or lose any of my reporting tools—two cameras, several lenses, a tape recorder, pens, and notepad—I shadowed doctors and nurses spending their vacations working twelve-hour days in ill-equipped hospitals, operating on children who should have been operated on years earlier—and would have been if the war hadn't prevented it. The doctors and nurses worked as long as they could during the two-week trip and operated on eighteen children. (There were twenty-six on the list, but a few got sick, one canceled, and one died before the team arrived.) All volunteers, the doctors and nurses awed me with their focus, their skill, and their willingness to spend the hours they weren't in surgery answering my questions over *pivo* (beer).

To me, the most inspiring kind of journalism requires great commitment from the journalist. Like good doctors, good journalists make sacrifices. They work long hours, do independent research, and spend time with the people they're trying to understand. For a pediatrician, a twenty-minute visit is better than a ten-minute one. For a journalist, a month-long immersion into someone else's life is better than a two-hour interview.

Our society is obsessed with doctors—we call on them at birth and death and every significant medical event in between—but rarely do we consider the personal challenges that doctors-to-be face. They are often ordinary people who have taken on an extraordinary challenge. Their motivations, I suspected, were far more interesting than many of us know from popular culture, with its fixation on television series about doctors. The first television doctor show I watched regularly as a child was *M.A.S.H.* After college, on Thursday nights I made sure to tune into *ER,* the doctors-on-adrenaline drama that often left me too wired for sleep. I first considered a project on medical students in the spring of 2005, after watching some of the first season of *Grey's Anatomy,* a hospital show focusing on the personal lives of interns whom, because of their poor decisions, you wouldn't trust to remove a plantar wart. Regardless of the quality of the writing, acting, and videography in these medical-themed shows, the doctor characters always drive the narratives. They are brilliant (even borderline miracle workers) but flawed. Despite their good looks, they are dedicated to medicine, which gives them nobility despite all the cheating they do on their spouses, all the drugs they take, and all the other transgressions that would lose the audience's sympathies if they were stars of shows focusing on lawyers, teachers, or journalists.

What keeps all the characters going is their love for medicine—for helping people get better after bloody school bus crashes and hospital hostage crises. I suspected that real medical students don't enter the field just to help people. There are many professions dedicated to helping people, few of which require the training commitment doctors make: two years of practically living in lecture halls and small study groups, learning biochemistry, histology, pharmacology, and every other "ology" one needs to know to practice medicine; another year learning every major medical service on the wards; several months spent dissecting a whole human body; and months more of original medical research resulting in a thesis. This training must be followed by three to five years of residency and, for many, additional years of fellowships. This is what is required to learn the science behind diagnosing illness and the art of treating patients.

One question, from then–assistant dean of admissions Dr. Lena Mehta, surprised me. She wanted to know if I would tell them if a student was in danger of committing suicide. I later learned that depression is relatively common among medical students. Medical educators worry about their students' mental states much more than, say, journalism educators do. According to a 2005 *New England Journal of Medicine* report, "White Coat, Mood Indigo—Depression in Medical School," medical students are more prone to depression than others their age because of the emotional and academic strain involved in becoming a doctor.

I believe in the fly-on-the-wall style of reporting—observe the present and don't do anything that might change the future. I had to think about Mehta's question before responding. Narrative journalist Anne Hull has described the ethical dilemmas that inevitably arise when a journalist can solve the problems of her subjects but chooses not to. While she was reporting on a poor family recently cut off from welfare benefits, their baby spiked a fever. After a while, it became clear that they needed to get her to the hospital, but they had no gas for their car. They kept looking at Hull, whose rental car was in the driveway, but she didn't offer to drive them, opting instead to see how they got themselves out of their predicament. Finally, the father pawned his shotgun for gas money, and they drove the baby to the hospital, where she recovered.

In "A Dilemma of Immersive Journalism," Hull explained she would have driven the family to the hospital if the baby's condition had become dire, but most of the time, journalists must not influence the stories unfolding around them. I agree with Hull. I decided I too would watch as the students solved their own problems. But if I thought a student was contemplating suicide, I would definitely tell the deans.

My time with the deans passed quickly, and I became more relaxed the less I talked. I had done all I could at that point—relayed my intentions and convinced them of my curiosity. After they stopped firing questions at me, the dean with the stylish glasses gave his blessing. He told me I would be reporting during the same year the school transitioned to a new curriculum, one that melded the goals of medical education and public health. This transition—given the major technological and scientific changes over the past few decades—was long overdue.

The current model of American medical education was established at the beginning of the previous century after the Carnegie Foundation for the Advancement of Teaching dispatched educator Abraham Flexner to each of the nation's 155 medical schools. Flexner's groundbreaking report, issued in 1910, criticized medical schools for their low standards and urged reform. The report fueled an upheaval in medical education, which resulted in medical schools becoming affiliated with universities, faculty working on original research, and students being taught in both labs and clinical settings. Although Case did pioneer another then-heralded curriculum change in 1952, the current evolution would be bigger—revolutionary, even.

I thought Horwitz and the deans were taking a huge risk. They had no way of knowing how things would turn out. Maybe if I were asking for access to a law school or a business school during a curricular "revolution," I would have been turned down. Why risk looking bad during a transition year? I'd think the administrators would want to make sure the curriculum worked before letting a journalist loose to write about it. But the gatekeepers in this case weren't just educators. They were doctors. One thing I've learned over the five years I spent reporting this story is that medicine is an imperfect science often practiced by perfectionists. As the author Atul Gawande has pointed out, there's a gap between what doctors know and what they aim for.

A general surgeon at the Brigham and Women's Hospital in Boston and a staff writer at the *New Yorker,* Gawande wrote his first book, *Complications,* while still a surgical resident. That was tricky. Doctors and hospitals don't like their shortcomings to be publicized—especially by one of their own. But Gawande found that "Even when my colleagues from work have disagreed with what I've written, they have been constructive and engaged and have held nothing against me. We are all, I've found, in the process of trying to understand how much of what we do is good, how much of it can be better."

Better, in fact, is the title of Gawande's second book. And though I am not a doctor, I am envious of the culture of responsibility that medicine tries to perpetuate. At academic hospitals, doctors gather once a week to explain why they made a particular call or prescribed a specific course of action that led to a grave unexpected consequence. These conversations can't be used in a court of law, so they tend to be frank discussions where mistakes can be divulged and reviewed and learned from. I would welcome a journalistic equivalent of morbidity and mortality conferences at news outlets and magazines. I have no doubt that if journalists had a place to talk about their own questionable calls without fear of legal retribution, we would be producing better journalism. What about lawyers, business executives, and educators? Is there any profession that wouldn't benefit from this kind of practice?

I left Horwitz's office feeling elated. To follow doctors-to-be during their training would be fascinating even during an average year—following them during a transitional year would give the piece some news heft. But it didn't take long for the worry to set in. I knew the next sell after the deans would be harder. I'd need to find a few students who would allow me into their lives and agree to speak with me regularly and follow them through what would probably be the most difficult period of their young lives.

On June 30, 2005, I wrote a letter to all incoming medical students. "From orientation to final exams, I will be there, observing and asking questions. As you're learning about medicine, I'll be learning about what it's like to be a doctor-in-training. As students of science, you know it's impossible to witness events without changing them in some way. The mere presence of an outsider can affect things. But it's my intention to be as unobtrusive as possible, to document the joys and challenges of this year through your eyes." In the letter, I asked students to initial the form in one place if they were interested in participating in the story, and in another place if they were not. I never asked to see the forms, though the public affairs director did tell me that few indicated they would not be interested in participating. I figured I'd wait until the semester began to start scouting for subjects. I explained the *what* in the letter but only a little of the *how:* I'd talk with three or four students (the main characters of my story) about once a week, interview others occasionally and attend events where I would be able to provide firsthand descriptions. With reporting, as with motherhood, you can only plan so much. You have to be present and be flexible. Sources you plan to turn into characters on the page often surprise you; sometimes they get so used to you they come to need you. Reporters are often (and sometimes unknowingly) "on call" for their subjects. They want us to witness things in their lives. I look forward to this happening, even though it can lead to some ethically difficult situations. In the letter, I told the students I planned to go to classes and clinical settings, but I'd need much more than access; I'd need their trust.

I thought the letter might improve my chances of finding willing subjects when I introduced myself at orientation. They wouldn't see me as some novice interloper but as a serious interloper, someone intensely interested in reporting what they were going through to a general-interest audience. I guessed that over four years they'd get tired of answering the question "What is medical school like?" I hoped they'd send my articles to friends and relatives who wanted to know.

On August 11, 2005, three days before the White Coat Ceremony, the class of 2009 gathered together for the first time in the main lecture hall. They were a diversely wardrobed group in khakis, jeans, ball caps, and spaghetti straps, sitting wrist-to-wrist and knee-to-knee, mostly behind faculty and administrators in white coats in the front rows. Dean Horwitz walked around in front of them, quoting William Butler Yeats ("Education is not the filling of a pail, but the lighting of a fire"), moving back toward the podium occasionally, reluctantly, not unlike a pinball when gravity first overtakes it, coaxing it back toward the paddles. "You are the most qualified group in the history of the medical school," the dean assured them. "You're extraordinarily well qualified for medical school."

In what seemed like a competitive way to start off a noncompetitive pass-fail year, the dean had the students stand up and share their names and undergraduate institutions. Graduates of Stanford and Harvard stood near those of Northwestern and University of Michigan, who stood near graduates of Westminster College and Wayne State. No matter where they came from or how they got here, years of study in an incredibly rigorous professional orientation awaited them, and Horwitz kicked it off with a simple round of applause from the faculty, building up the students' confidence before the work tore it down.

He told them about Case's great tradition of producing excellent physicians, a tradition that dates back to 1843, when Case's predecessor, the Medical Department of Western Reserve College, also known as Cleveland Medical College, opened. American medical education was the worst in the industrialized world back then, and if you really wanted to learn medicine, you had to go to Europe. But the Cleveland school was more advanced than most.

As the decades wore on, the college continued to excel beyond most of its peer institutions. While other schools were shamed by Flexner's skewering 1910 report, Flexner himself complimented the medical training at Western Reserve. In terms of quality, Flexner wrote in a letter to Western Reserve University president Charles F. Thwing, only Johns Hopkins surpassed it. But Thomas Hale Ham, Western Reserve's future chairman of the Committee on Medical Education, said the department, like most medical departments of the time, put the needs of the departments first. "The student inherited the departmental research, the excellence and complexity[,] but was often lost as an individual and as a member of community medicine," he said.

Hale Ham held strong opinions on this, and he helped orchestrate the next big change in medical education in 1952. At that time, Western Reserve drew national attention for pioneering a new curriculum that addressed some critical problems with traditional medical education: students feeling overwhelmed by the crush of information, memorization being stressed over analytical skills, and the separation of basic (the first two years) and clinical sciences (the last two). Hale Ham wrote about the reasons for this evolution in *The Student as Colleague: Medical Education Experience at Case Western Reserve,* published in 1976.

"Because of concern over the overwhelming mass of departmental material presented to the student along with a growing awareness that the true needs of the learner had been forgotten, the faculty of the School of Medicine at Western Reserve University began in 1946 to plan a new program," he wrote. The new curriculum signaled a new era in medical education, one "marked by interdepartmental teaching of medical knowledge through subject committees; by the creation of multidisciplinary laboratories for individual student use; by student participation in patient care during the first year of medical training; by new methods of instruction; and, basic to the program's entire development, by instructor treatment of the student as a client and at the same time a colleague."

Dean Joseph T. Wearn started having students do clinical work during the first year, treated students as colleagues, and integrated basic and clinical sciences. Instead of teaching individual subjects—for instance, the pathology of the whole body covered in one course—Western Reserve faculty taught organ systems. Students learned everything about the heart when they studied the cardiovascular system, including its biology, histology, and pharmacology. Other medical schools then consulted the Western Reserve model in revising their own curricula.

In 1967, Western Reserve University merged with the Case Institute of Technology to become Case Western Reserve University, and the medical school's reputation remains strong today. To underscore this, Horwitz told the students about the school's connections to eleven Nobel laureates and two U.S. surgeons general.

Other faculty members then took the floor to talk about more practical things—class pictures, computers, the curriculum roadmap. When Horwitz came back to the front of the lecture hall, he addressed the issue of professionalism. There was no drum roll or curtain rise, but the excitement in his voice hinted at his topic's importance with the subtlety of a trumpet blast. This took at least one student I spoke with later that day, Michael Norton, by surprise. He wondered, "What kind of fluff lecture is this?"

"Case traditions are embedded in the concept of professionalism," said Horwitz, who went on to break down its two fundamental components. The first resides in the personal. It's what makes doctors put their patients' needs ahead of their own, a "powerful, compelling, and overbearing" sense of personal responsibility. It's what makes them reject dinners, lunches, pens, and other gifts from the pharmaceutical industry, none of which are welcome at Case. The other component of professionalism resides in the profession, "a sense of collective responsibility." Together, doctors must maintain their commitment to quality health care and efficiency. The 45 million uninsured are *their* problem. The overuse, underuse, and misuse of medical technology? Those are also their problems, as are the inconsistencies in health-care outcomes based on race, ethnicity, and social status.

The class of 2009 is the most qualified group of students in the history of the medical school, he said. As the next generation of doctors, how are they going to solve these problems?

Norton was sitting next to me throughout this lecture, biting his nails.

I suspected his reasons for going into medicine didn't differ that much from the reasons of med students of previous generations. Because of *when* he entered medical school, however, he was going to be a guinea pig—or a "pioneer," depending on your perspective—which gave him something in common with the doctors-to-be of the early and mid-twentieth century, other periods of major change in medical education. Attention to the needs of the patients (with some help from Flexner) kicked off the first revolution in medical education in 1910, when great disparities in medical education resulted in great disparities in health care. The needs of the students grappling with a swelling amount of medical research and clinical demands drove the 1952 curriculum change. The needs of the community drove the 2006 one. Like his predecessors, Norton would learn pulmonology and neurology. He would be trained to identify a cancerous skin lesion and interpret an EKG. But through Case's integration of the studies of medicine and public health, he and the rest of the class of 2009 would also concern themselves much more with the health of the community, considering the social and behavioral contexts of illness.

To help initiate them into this new mind-set, Dr. Steven Ricanati challenged them to craft their own "document of professionalism." Ricanati was one of the school's four society deans. At Case, every incoming student was appointed to one of the four societies, named after prominent alumni and faculty: Emily Blackwell, who in 1854 became the third woman to earn a medical degree in the United States; Frederick C. Robbins, a Nobel Prize winner who helped develop a vaccine for polio; David Satcher, a former U.S. surgeon general; and Joseph Wearn, the former dean credited with improving medical education nationwide after the school's 1952 curriculum change. Since 2003, the deans of these four societies have advised students and provided social outlets, such as group dinners and movie nights.

Now, Ricanati can be a funny guy. He's the only society dean with a ponytail, and he had just told the new students that 10 percent of them would get married at the end of four years. (All four society deans are married to physicians.) When he told them they only had until the end of the day to finish writing the oath, I doubt I was the only one who thought he was joking. Surely, the students had all heard of the Hippocratic Oath, a statement of ethics composed in ancient Greece around 400 B.C. The students would have to recite a modern version at commencement. But write an original professionalism document on the first day of medical school orientation? Right. Perhaps they could also whip up a differential diagnosis on the side.

As is often the case in medicine, thankfully, the students would not be tackling something that seemed impossible by themselves. Ricanati had a plan: The students would break into groups of seven or eight, the same small groups they would meet with over the next eighteen months as part of a course called the Science of Clinical Practice. With faculty and fourth-year student helpers, each group would develop a list of bullet points reflecting their collective values. Representatives from each group would then meet to merge all their lists into one meaningful, succinct document of professionalism to be read—or performed—during the White Coat Ceremony. (According to the script provided to the Professionalism Workshop organizers, the first task for the student leaders was to decide on the format of the document. "Options include: Contract, Oath, Poem, Song, Dance, Narrative." No group I saw seriously considered a non-oath format, but that was my first indication there would be song and dance in the med students' future.)

What is professionalism? I doubted this was the question foremost in the mind of the average med student on orientation day. Many of them, including Millie Gentry, got through the first part as quickly as they could and went home. Others, including Marleny Franco, took it more seriously.

At 3:15 P.M., after all but eight of her classmates had gone home, Franco still stood at a podium in a darkened conference room, typing on a laptop computer in front of a large screen displaying the list of values from which her class's "Oath of Professionalism" ought to spring. The deadline was 4 P.M.

To Franco, this was not a meaningless academic exercise. It was important. She knew what she wanted in that oath: a line about a commitment to alleviate health-care disparities based on language, race, and culture. While she was still an undergraduate, Franco did asthma research in Latino communities and was shocked by how little the parents knew about their children's disease. They told her things they'd never tell a research assistant who didn't speak their language.

"You know what it's like in the DR," one parent said, mentioning the home remedy of "lizard in boiled milk" for asthma. Franco, who was born in the Dominican Republic, had never heard of such a thing. She doubted the parent would have been honest about this to a doctor who didn't speak Spanish.

The other students suggested big-picture concepts as well: honesty, humility, and patience, among them. The screen was filled with words, but the students hadn't written even one line of the oath. "This is the hard part," society dean Elizabeth McKinley told them empathetically. "How do you get it down to a couple of lines? It's hard."

At 3:36 P.M., they had three lines. At 3:40 P.M., they asked for an extension. The dean, now considerably less empathetic, just said, "You've got to get this done."

"It's nice to be sensitive and all that," Ricanati said. "But patients want to be fixed. That keeps getting pushed down."

Someone brought up "equity of care" and mentioned that it had been controversial in an earlier group discussion. Someone else brought up "passion." They kept editing as they wrote, trying to weave in all their points.

Then Microsoft Word crashed, and there was a collective "Noooooooooo!"

Luckily, one student had an undergraduate degree in computer science. She got the document back. The breakthrough came soon after that. Two good lines: "Today we begin a lifetime of responsibilities to our patients, our society, our colleagues, and ourselves. We will strive towards honesty, integrity, open-mindedness and compassion."

The students didn't make the deadline, but they finished. Confronted with no resistance at all, Franco landed her views in the penultimate point: "We will provide impartial and compassionate care without discrimination and judgment." It was a small accomplishment, and someone later changed the wording. But the sentiment stood, and she was proud of the document. At the time, she didn't even know I was planning to ask her to be one of my subjects. She just knew someone from her class would read the oath at the White Coat Ceremony. It would reflect on them, she said. On her. It wasn't just a bunch of words; it was a glimpse of the doctors they would become one day.

Oath of Professionalism

August 11, 2005

Today we begin a lifetime of responsibilities to our patients, our society, our profession, and ourselves.

To our patients, we promise to:

- Strive for mastery of medical knowledge and clinical skills
- Respect their individuality, beliefs, privacy, and autonomy
- Empower them through encouragement and education
- Communicate with warmth and clarity
- Recognize their physical, social, and emotional health, and
- Relentlessly advocate for their best interests

To our society, we promise:

- A committed effort toward quality healthcare for all
- Leadership in eliminating health disparities
- Dedicated to medical and scientific progress, and
- Efficient, justifiable use of influence and resources

To our profession, we promise to:

- Cooperate, collaborate, and respect one another
- Exemplify the ideals of the practice of medicine, and
- Uphold the integrity of medicine by promoting accountability

In these pursuits, we will strive towards honesty, integrity, open-mindedness and compassion. We will temper our confidence with a humble acknowledgement of our limitations. We commit to self-improvement and life-long learning.

With these words, we hereby devote ourselves to a lifetime of improving the health of patients and society.

The White Coat Ceremony

Marleny Franco

In Reinberger Chamber Hall, the staging area for the White Coat Ceremony, Marleny Franco imagined herself falling off the stage, arms flailing, face aghast. She should not have worn heels today; she wasn't used to heels. She wore them because she was twenty-four and a little vain, because her mother and her father were in the audience, because all the new friends she'd just made were there, because the professors she wanted to impress were there, because though she was an Ivy League graduate and her mother's *bella genio* (beautiful genius), she wanted to look good, damn good, in her short white coat. It awaited her on a rack in the middle of the stage, in fine company, surrounded by other short white coats, one for each of her classmates at the Case Western Reserve University School of Medicine, ranked number 20 (out of 143 accredited medical schools) in 2006 by *U.S. News and World Report.* Close to 5,000 applicants wanted a Case Med coat this year. Only Franco and 166 others got one.

No one had tried on his or her coat yet, and in addition to worrying about a slip off the stage, Franco, who tells people to pronounce her first name by putting "Marx" and "Lennon" together, worried about her coat fitting properly. She knew she had four years to fill it out, but, again, she's a little vain. She's also a lot sensitive to what distinguishes her from her classmates: she is a Latina—and poor. Her parents divorced when she was nine, and then her mother moved her and her sister from the Dominican Republic to the Dominican projects of Boston. Because her mother couldn't speak English, she couldn't be a nurse as she was in the Dominican Republic. Instead, she became a janitor. When Franco's father followed them to the city five years later, he went from working in a bank to working as a carpenter.

Franco's mother encouraged her daughter's curiosity about all things medical, a curiosity Franco can trace back to when she was five or six. After school let out, she'd pass the afternoons in her mother's Santo Domingo hospital. Instead of playing quietly in the waiting room as she was told, she would wander into trauma bays and treatment rooms. And before her mother's nurse friends could intercept her, she saw all sorts of forbidden things. The more blood and gore she encountered, the more interested she became. In America, Franco became *la hija que sabe Ingles* (the daughter who knows English), the one who filled out medical forms for her mom's friends and Spanish-speaking strangers at the local health clinic. Franco excelled in school, especially in science and math, testing into the Boston Latin Academy in seventh grade. In high school, she sought out more advanced science training and did college-level research at Harvard Medical School under the guidance of scientists there.

She studied community health at Brown University and researched childhood asthma for two years after college. One of her bosses was Dr. Bob Klein, a pediatric asthma expert who became her mentor. Franco was accepted at seven medical schools, eventually narrowing her choice down to either the University of Pittsburgh or Case. Money was an important consideration, and Pitt gave her more grants. But Case impressed her during Second Look Weekend, when those accepted are invited back to spend time with students, faculty, and alumni. She dined at the gorgeous home of a Case faculty member and stayed out with other prospective students and Dean Ralph Horwitz until 2 A.M. (Franco saw Pitt's dean for maybe ten minutes.) It was a Case student who told her about the Jack Kent Cooke Foundation scholarship program. The foundation awards a small number of graduate students as much as $50,000 for tuition, living expenses, and other educational costs annually for up to six years.

"You will get the scholarship," the student told her, "and you will come to Case."

Although Franco wasn't so confident, she filled out the enormous application and waited. Three months passed. She assumed she didn't get the scholarship, but she couldn't stop thinking about Case. Things felt good there. People reached out to her, even the dean. She saw more faces like hers, but they all seemed to come from more money. It scared her to think about how much she'd have to borrow to attend Case. For her first year, tuition would cost $37,944 and living expenses another $15,108. Even with some grants, Franco still had to sign a promissory loan for $41,116. A few days after signing, however, she found out she could cancel the loan. The Cooke scholarship was hers.

She told me about the scholarship during our first interview, at Presti's, a café in Little Italy near campus. She declined a coffee because she'd recently given up caffeine. Franco mentioned right away that her minority status had no bearing on her getting the scholarship. The foundation's mission is to help "high-achieving, lower-income students" in high school, college, and graduate school. She was sure I'd made a common assumption—that she got the scholarship because she is a minority—and she was right. Yet she didn't hold that against me. Our differences were obvious: I'm white, the product of a mostly suburban upbringing. My ethnicity resides in my name and in the dishes my family still cooks, and I'd never felt like a minority. Growing up, I visited all white doctors, mostly middle-aged men with whom I spent very little time and shared nothing I wouldn't tell my mother. Our misunderstandings had nothing to do with language or culture.

Even though Franco and I come from different backgrounds, we talked easily with one another. My story would be a way to tell her story, she said. She wanted to show other immigrant kids they can get into medical school too.

After the procession to Severance Hall, Franco took her place in the audience. On the stage in front of her stood rows of deans, including medical school dean Horwitz and Dr. Eric Topol, provost of the Cleveland Clinic Lerner College of Medicine, a collaborative five-year MD program of Case and the Clinic in its second year of existence. With Horwitz and Topol stood the society deans, the students' advisers and confidants. All the deans wore long white coats with red flowers in their lapels.

The hall was noisy with chatter and camera flashes, the students fidgeting in their seats, craning their necks to see their families, smiling just-met-you smiles to their neighbors.

"Wow!" Horwitz exclaimed from the podium, signaling, *Quiet!* He assured the crowd that these students had "stunning" backgrounds. They came from all over the country. Fifteen grew up abroad. Most had research experience. "Thank God we didn't have to compete with them for admission," Horwitz said.

After a few other speeches and more applause, the keynote speaker, society dean Robert Haynie, approached the podium. Haynie has presence, but it's a different sort of presence from that of an actor or an athlete—or even the other doctors on the stage. He is lanky and long armed, gray haired, and effortlessly emphatic. When he was growing up in the 1950s, there weren't many black chemists. Haynie would become one. His second advanced degree is in medicine. He is also a father of seven, a fighter of obesity and hypertension, and an ad-lib storyteller of the first order.

He said he was going to tell them about wearing the white coat. But first he wanted to tell them about a time he took it off.

"You never judge a man who stands in a pool of tranquility," he began, paraphrasing Martin Luther King. "You only judge a man when he stands in a pathway of adversity." On one of Haynie's pathways, he thought he might lose his daughter. Tracie was nineteen at the time, a college student on spring break in Atlanta. She was standing in line outside a nightclub when someone brandished a gun. Someone else abruptly backed up his car, pinning Tracie against a truck, transecting her liver and rupturing both her hepatic vein and inferior vena cava.

The fidgety audience quieted down. Franco had never been in a concert hall so quiet.

Haynie continued. He said he flew down to Georgia Baptist Hospital and went straight to the surgical intensive care unit. He was sitting in the waiting room, tears rolling down his face as he thought of his daughter's injuries, any one of which could kill her. Then Haynie spotted a picture hanging crooked on the wall, and he was seized by an absurd thought, especially for a man with doctorates in chemistry and medicine. *Maybe if I straighten the picture, Tracie will get better.* When he walked to the wall to straighten it—a photograph of twin brothers walking on the beach—the inscription under it made him pause. It said one of the boys in the picture had died when he was three years old. His parents donated his organs so some other children could live. After reading that, Haynie knew what he needed to do—give permission for his daughter's organs to be harvested.

Where is this going? Franco worried. She was emotional enough without this story.

Back in the waiting room, Haynie continued, a woman who had just lost her sixteen-year-old grandson approached him. "Son, I know you're in pain," she said. "Do you mind if I pray for you?"

Haynie was floored by the gesture, by how someone suffering so much could focus on trying to alleviate the suffering of a stranger. She pressed a small cross into the palm of his hand. When he got home, he put it in the pocket of his white coat.

The tears were starting. Franco could feel them. *Damn it, Haynie.*

"I can't end the story there," the society dean said in closing. "Tracie, stand up."

Franco joined in the thunderous applause at seeing Haynie's daughter stand up in the balcony. His message to the new med students, though he never said it directly, was this: You must take off your white coat sometimes. Don't just be a doctor. Be a husband, a wife, a father, a mother. Let those other roles improve your doctoring.

There are three Posits of Haynie: (1) Have a family life. (2) Attempt to make a lot of money. (3) Be a good doctor. You can only do two out of three, he said. To pick the right two, the coat must go on, and it must come off. Know when to wear it on your pathways of adversity. Know when to carry your crucifixes in your pocket.

Millie Gentry

Millie Gentry wasn't listening to the White Coat Ceremony speeches, not really. While Horwitz and others were praising the students in the class of 2009 for their brilliance and potential, she was thinking about how to escape them. She was wondering what kind of modeling scene existed in Cleveland, about whether she'd be able to get a job. She wanted some extra money. She wanted friends outside the med school. She wanted to travel.

I first met Gentry in Reinberger Chamber Hall just before the procession to Severance Hall. She arrived late, after most everyone else had been seated. She had long, dark hair then, with bangs that refused to behave, and she wore a strapless dress with a classy floral pattern with lots of red. I introduced myself as she was rushing down the aisle. Despite her lateness, she stopped to talk with me. I learned later that strangers were always approaching Gentry—she is striking, statuesque, and half Taiwanese on her mother's side—and she enjoys making new connections. She was curious about what I was doing at the ceremony and very nice, too. The other students I approached were all nice but distracted. Gentry wanted to talk. I asked her how she felt about getting her white coat, and she surprised me with an answer that was far more candid than the one anyone else had given me. "I just want to go home and get some sheets," she said. "I've been sleeping on an air mattress. It's really uncomfortable."

Gentry was twenty-four and from Florence, Arizona, a small town an hour outside Phoenix with a high teen-pregnancy rate. Her parents ran a grocery store there, and her high school classmates still didn't believe she was in med school. It's just not something many girls from Florence did. But they didn't often pursue biology degrees at Smith College in Northampton, Massachusetts, either. Or work as a model. Or go to Taiwan alone to take a job teaching English. Gentry told me these things later, along with how her mind rambled during the speeches. It intrigued me that she had great in-the-moment interest in a stranger asking her lame reporter questions, but she had no patience for the ceremonial start to what would be the most challenging four years of her life.

I promised to bug her often, to give her an opportunity to talk to someone outside labs and classrooms. She became, as I suspected from our first meeting, the least reliable of my subjects, the one who induced the worst writer's block. She didn't fit into any preconceived notion of what a medical student should be. She wasn't driven. She wasn't out to save the world. She talked to me about yoga, running, socializing, and fashion. Our conversations became games, each one a tug of war. She wanted to talk about life; I wanted to talk about school. I gave her a little about my one-year-old daughter (she loves children), my vacation, the dinners I cooked. She gave me a little about how horrible the last test was for her. I wanted her hopes and dreams. She wanted restaurant recommendations. She sent me a gift card for my birthday. I sent it back.

Even at the White Coat Ceremony, Gentry already felt distanced from her classmates. She said they were mostly "gunners," students who wanted to ace everything in medical school, even during the first pass-fail year. She was at the other end of the spectrum, haunted by the memory of three garbage bags overflowing with notes, papers, and exams from her undergraduate years. While other people were making friends, meeting significant others, joining clubs, learning other languages, and just living, Gentry was studying hard, filling up those bags. She was determined not to spend another four years of her life with her head buried in books. Instead, she vowed to bake, to shop, and to go out on weeknights. While other students adopted a succeed-at-all-costs attitude toward medical school, she had already decided—even before she received her white coat—to embark on what may be an impossible pursuit: to become a medical student with a life.

Michael Norton

At the White Coat Ceremony, Michael Norton sat up front. He looked like many other young men wearing dress shirts and ties, but he also sported the laid-back demeanor of a guy whose comic hero is Dr. Cox from the NBC sitcom *Scrubs*. Unlike some of his colleagues who'd spent the previous evening partying—drinking beer and spray-painting the Case logo, a rising sun, on a table—Norton wasn't tired or hung over. Two of his dreams were coming true at about the same time: he was entering the practice of medicine, and in less than two months, he was going to become a father.

Norton was awed by his colleagues' intelligence, not envious of their social lives. He'd heard med school was like returning to high school in that respect. Being Mormon, Norton has the church to fulfill his social needs. When he and his wife, Kate, moved from Utah to Cleveland a few weeks earlier, they instantly had friends—and not just why-don't-you-come-over-for-dinner-sometime friends. The Nortons' new friends from the Church of Jesus Christ of Latter-day Saints helped them get out of the sketchy East Cleveland apartment they'd leased over the Internet and found them a nice duplex ten minutes from school.

Norton's father, Bryan, told me his son never went through the fireman stage. He never wanted to be cowboy or an astronaut, only a doctor. At four years old, Norton became fascinated with stethoscopes. By the time he was eight, he owned a microscope, a telescope, and a chemistry set. At eleven, he earned a Boy Scout merit badge in atomic energy. Academically, everything Norton has done—including the advanced placement science courses he took in high school and the microbiology major he completed in college—he's done to get into medical school. He'd made it here. Now what? He hadn't thought much beyond actually getting to medical school, about what would happen to him here. He'd heard you get 500 pages of reading a day, and that he'd be lucky to squeeze in four hours of sleep a night.

When I first asked Norton why he'd always wanted to be a doctor, he answered over the course of several conversations and e-mails. Adding to his childhood fascination, medical school seemed like the logical next step after majoring in microbiology at Brigham Young University and working on screening tests for genetic mutations that predispose people to breast, ovarian, and colorectal cancer at Myriad Genetic Laboratories in Utah. It seemed like the type of work that would suit him personally—few other professions would enable him to use his knowledge and skills to improve people's lives every day. But he also felt it was his responsibility. "As I've grown up, I've come to realize that there is an enormous amount of suffering in the world and that some individuals receive far more than what might be considered their 'fair share,'" he wrote in one e-mail. "I've been blessed with a sound body and mind (though my friends and family might argue about the latter), and I've developed an acute sense of responsibility to help those who may not be so fortunate."

For our first substantial interview, I met Norton at his rented duplex. Kate, who was twenty-one and two months away from becoming a mother, joined us at the kitchen table. She was smart and blonde and looked exactly her age. Her baby belly seemed strapped onto her otherwise slight frame, but she didn't seem worn down by the major changes in her life: the pregnancy, a husband starting medical school, or the move across the country. Kate liked to talk, and she was easy to talk with—present, focused, and calm.

Norton and Kate met at Brigham Young University outside a testing center. She was studying linguistics, a degree she completed in three years. They were engaged two months after they met and married five months after becoming engaged. They had a reception in Kate's family's backyard, complete with a fountain her father and brother began building almost immediately after Norton proposed. From our first meeting, I learned some things about the Nortons that I'd expected. They spent a lot of time with other Mormons. They prayed before they ate, even with visitors present. Kate took care of things at home, freeing Norton to study more than non-married med students who have to do their own cooking and laundry. Other things surprised me, including how much Norton looked to his wife to provide more detail to the stories he told. Kate often interjected her own insights into the conversation, sometimes disagreeing with Norton and even cutting him off. I've known plenty of wives to cut off their husbands mid-sentence, but Norton's reaction was different. He seemed fine with it, completely unfazed.

Soon after I asked Norton to be in my magazine story, he sent me an e-mail expressing surprise that I "chose" him. He figured it was because he was different from many of the other students. He was married. He was twenty-five, whereas many students go to medical school right out of college. He also thought it might be because he liked chatting. "So about me and chatting . . . I've felt bad ever since Friday because I was afraid I talked your ear off until you were completely sick of me. I was diagnosed with attention deficit hyperactivity disorder when I was very young (I think it was before I even started kindergarten). One of the lesser-known but extremely obnoxious tendencies of ADHD kids and adults is a tendency to chattiness and rambling, and I'm well aware that I have that problem quite often. Long story short, don't hesitate to tell me to can it if I won't shut up. I won't be offended; in fact, I'll probably have been telling myself to be quiet for a while already."

So much is written about what doctors should know, how they should act, and the processes they go through to improve health care. Sure, it helps if a doctor has a good bedside manner, but does it matter if he yammers on too much? Medical school began with a lecture on professionalism. No one talked about personality. From Norton, I expected to learn about what it's like to be a medical student with a family. I learned that he would also be teaching me about what it's like to be a medical student with ADHD. He didn't worry about missing parties; he worried about missing social cues. Tests and procedures only tell a doctor so much. He would have to learn to talk to people and, more important, to listen.

•◆◆•

One by one, the students were called to the stage to receive their coats. Franco walked to where her society dean, Dr. Charles Kent Smith, waited to help her, the clicking of her heels audible throughout the concert hall. She was thinking of Harry Potter, about the similarities between the heads of houses in their long robes and the deans in their long coats, the students looking to them for guidance. Norton beamed, looking for his family in the audience: his pregnant wife, both his parents. It was Gentry, the model, who slipped on the stage. Just then, her father snapped a picture, capturing her struggle to regain her balance, white coat billowing, framing her strapless dress.

The Science

On the first day of biochemistry, E301 was packed and noisy with the trills of laptops turning on and the excited chatter of eager students. Students had styled their hair, fully applied their makeup, and ironed their shirts; this level of personal grooming would drop considerably by the end of the week. The lecture-hall seats, arranged in an ascending stadium-seating pattern, were secured to the floor close enough to each other that you could smell the coffee of the person next to you, hear him shifting his weight or biting his pen cap. How motivated these students will have be, I thought, to weather such distractions for hours every day.

William Merrick, biochemistry committee chair, a mustachioed man with arched Jack Nicholson–like eyebrows, stood at the podium. Students should consider themselves "physicians in training," he said. They should "act accordingly," "behave professionally," and dress for class as if they were going to see patients. "We don't want to have you caught in the transition between panty raids and diagnosing cancer," he said. After this brief introduction, he ceded the floor to a faculty member teaching the thermodynamics of energy metabolism.

Franco was there, as she was almost every day, motivated by fear. Franco was not a gunner; she just wanted to survive biochemistry. As many as one-third of first-year students fail that committee. At least that's what some second-year students were saying. It's really only about 10 percent, Merrick told me. But one-third was what the first-years had heard, solidifying biochem's reputation as the boot camp of medical school. Unlike Mike Norton, who studied biochemistry extensively as an undergraduate and for whom this course would be mostly review, Franco was a community health major in college. She quickly found it impossible to keep up with the reading on the body's chemicals and processes. Students were holed up in E301 for several hours a day getting molecules and biochemical pathways thrown at them, trying to follow lessons prepared by a parade of PhDs wielding pointers. Beta oxidation, energy metabolism, ionic configurations of amino acids. All the new nomenclature and methodology. It was a grind. She felt as if she would never, ever learn it all.

But no one can learn it all. Trying to do so is one of the biggest mistakes new medical students make. They think they can study in medical school the same way they studied in college. Many of them are used to acing exams with minimal or last-minute effort. But in med school, cramming doesn't work. There's too much material. Traditionally, students spent the first two years of medical school learning the science: the normal during the first year, and the abnormal during the second. But the amount of medical knowledge is exploding. What doctors think they know about something changes quickly with new research. So medical students are taught the importance of becoming "lifelong learners." This is the only way, educators contend, that doctors can keep up with the pace of medical research. Just look at the number of journals and citations in MEDLINE, a database containing more than 18 million references to articles in both national and international journals on life sciences, with a concentration in biomedicine. According to the National Library of Medicine's Detailed Indexing Statistics, there were 5,394 journals in MEDLINE in 2010, up from 3,484 in 1995. The number of citations has grown from 1,098,015 in 1970 to 17,641,559 in 2009. Biomedical was the largest subject area in the active peer-reviewed journals cataloged by STM, the International Association of Scientific, Technical and Medical Publishers, accounting for 30 percent of its 25,400 titles in early 2009.

Even in the late 1950s, first-year students felt overwhelmed by the expanding body of medical knowledge. The tremendous amount of material was "the new and most pressing problem faced by all students in their freshman year," and they called it "the overload," wrote a group of sociologists who studied medical student culture at the University of Kansas Medical School and later published their report in the 1961 book *Boys in White*. Exams were the way the faculty determined if the students had learned the material, and students were terrified of them. There was little direction from the faculty on what material was the most important. Fifty years after the University of Kansas study, students were still complaining about the quantity of the material, the lack of clarity about what to study, and the difficulty of the exams.

At Case, subjects were taught in "committees," courses designed and taught by groups of faculty members. Biochem was where it became obvious to Franco that the curriculum was in transition. To help make time for students to complete a research thesis, material that used to be taught in the second year was now being taught in the first. As a result, the biochem committee had to compress the material that it used to teach over five weeks into three and a half—warp speed to Franco.

She studied so late at night that she sometimes slept through her alarm. When she made it to class, she sometimes fell asleep, and she wasn't the only one. Students were falling asleep all over the lecture hall. Franco started drinking caffeinated beverages again. She stopped going to class after a while and instead watched the lectures, which were all recorded, on her computer at double speed, stopping and rewinding parts that confused her. She went to the reviews twice a week when she had specific questions. Otherwise, she found them unhelpful.

While I understood the reasons for the new curriculum, I was confused by how the school planned to make better physicians out of students by shortening the teaching time. I sat through a biochemistry session with the students, and it just seemed like the professor was giving a lecture, the traditional method of instructing first-year students on biochemistry. With the new curriculum, however, he had less time. I talked with Dr. Terry Wolpaw, a longtime medical educator and associate dean for curricular affairs. She told me it was not the amount of time but the effectiveness of the teaching that mattered.

"You can't teach it all in twenty-four months," she explained. "You can't teach it all in ten years." Reducing the amount of "passive" learning, such as lectures, was a trend in medical education and one feature of the new curriculum. In 2006, first-year students would carry much more of the educational burden in additional small-group sessions, which would include more integration of subject matter. But, as with any colossal curricular change, not all the professors were onboard with the dean. Of the students who would be shaped by this curriculum, one instructor told me, "I wonder what sort of doctors they'll be."

That first week of biochem, Franco's initial praise for the school's public health focus morphed into frustration. She no longer wanted to hear about big-picture curriculum changes; she wanted more time to study biochem. Second-year students had almost twice as much time to learn nearly the same amount of material. She learned that the all-night cramming she had done during her undergraduate years didn't work in medical school. She couldn't miss even one day. She stopped playing racquetball because she couldn't justify the amount of time it took her away from her work. She got so little sleep that she started nodding off in class. The week before their first major exam of medical school, Franco pulled several all-nighters at the school, sometimes napping in the lounges. She wasn't fully awake when the exam started at 8 A.M. on September 16. She began with the short-answer questions because the first one seemed easy. The second was harder, the third harder still. One question involved the process of cholesterol synthesis—something she had taught another student several hours earlier. But she couldn't remember it for the test. She fell asleep and awoke when her head hit her desk. She went to the bathroom and splashed water on her face. It didn't help her remember cholesterol synthesis. She worked on the multiple-choice section. At noon, she turned in her unfinished test.

Afterward, the student she'd helped understand cholesterol synthesis thanked her. She didn't tell him she had forgotten it herself. This was what she did remember: the orientation-week lecture about failing a committee, how the whole room went silent as the remediation process was explained. Franco knew that if she failed, she'd have to keep studying biochem while trying to learn the same new material as the rest of the class. Eventually she'd have to take another biochem test.

She walked over to her desk in the green room, one of the cube farms on the third floor. Taking a deep breath, she flipped open her laptop again and checked how she did on the multiple-choice section. It wasn't until after she had walked home and climbed the stairs to her room that she began to cry.

At Case, if a student fails one committee, he or she has to meet with the society dean and committee chair and take another test (or some other assessment determined by the committee chair). If students fail two committees in a three- or four-month block, they have to take the mastery exam, a cumulative test that covers every subject learned during that block—even those they've already passed. Franco failed two: biochem and pulmonology.

If she failed the mastery exam, she'd have to go before a faculty committee, which would determine what would happen next. The committee can require a student to take a leave of absence, repeat the year, or leave the school altogether. As the first-year students breaked for winter, Franco flew home to Boston for a week. The mastery exam she planned to take January 7 crowded most everything else out of her mind. But she didn't tell her parents about it. Every time her proud mother called her *mi bella genio,* she wanted to climb out of her skin. She did confide in Bob Klein, her "second father" and the doctor with whom she'd researched racial, cultural, and socioeconomic disparities among child asthmatics, but she downplayed the test as a mere annoyance. He and his wife held a gathering in her honor at their Providence, Rhode Island, home. They served baked chicken and sweet potatoes, two of her favorite foods. She smiled and schmoozed with the head of the lab where she used to work, one of her recommenders for the Jack Kent Cooke scholarship.

She felt like a fake. She worried about jeopardizing her scholarship. That, for her, would be the hardest thing to bear. She had exceeded people's expectations her whole life. Many kids who started where she did still lived in the ghetto. But she had proved that a poor Latina girl could get an Ivy League education and win a prestigious scholarship to medical school. For her, flunking out was unimaginable.

She flew back on Christmas Day and retreated to her deserted third-floor apartment on Hampshire Road, where she studied by herself for a solid week. Other students were taking the mastery exam, but she didn't know who. So she let word get around that she was taking it. And one by one, the others contacted her. A few days before the test, they formed a study group she dubbed "The Breakfast Club," after the 1985 movie about a group of high school students who bond over weekend detention.

As the exam approached, Franco's resolve grew. *They're not getting rid of me,* she decided. The night before the test on January 7, 2006, she actually slept. The next morning her stomach was settled and her mind clear.

About half of the test was essay questions and half was multiple choice. It was supposed to last four hours. But Franco's computer crashed three times during the exam, erasing her longest essay three times. She had tears in her eyes when the professor told her they could take an extra hour to finish. Four long days later, she found out she'd passed.

•◆◆•

At Case in 2006, not all first-year learning was as rigorous as biochemistry. Before that course, there was Fundamentals of Medical Decision-Making, which culminated with skits performed by the students in the main lecture hall. For her skit, Millie Gentry wore a halter top stuffed with toilet paper and a "Pam Anderson" nametag. It was not the most creative costume, but she hoped people would find it funny. Along with "Martha Stewart," "Naomi Judd," and, of course, "Tommy Lee," she planned to relay hepatitis C information in *Hollywood Squares* fashion. She scanned the audience quickly for her group and felt her stomach drop. The refrain *I feel really stupid right now* started running through her head. No one else from her group was wearing any sort of costume. Worse, no one laughed at hers.

The med students evaluated each other's public-awareness skits with laughter, not grades. Oompa Loompas hauled away the hopelessly confused in Willy Wonka's Happy Fun Time Alzheimer's Clinic. An *Austin Powers*–inspired ode to prostate-cancer screening starred the hysterically mismatched Norton and Franco (sporting an afro wig) as a married couple. A somewhat disturbing skit on lead testing drew laughs with a diaper-clad med student and songs that would have made Barney the purple dinosaur proud. All original. Gentry's skit was last on the chuckle meter, and her initial assessment was confirmed. Her classmates—the ones not in her group anyway—were gunners. She didn't fit in, and she kept trying to convince herself that she didn't care.

When a faculty member helping the students with their research said she hoped they would all win Nobel Prizes someday, Gentry said she'd rather work part time and have two kids and a minivan. The faculty member thought she was kidding. She wasn't. At the end of four years, she wanted to be a doctor, but she wanted to have a regular life too.

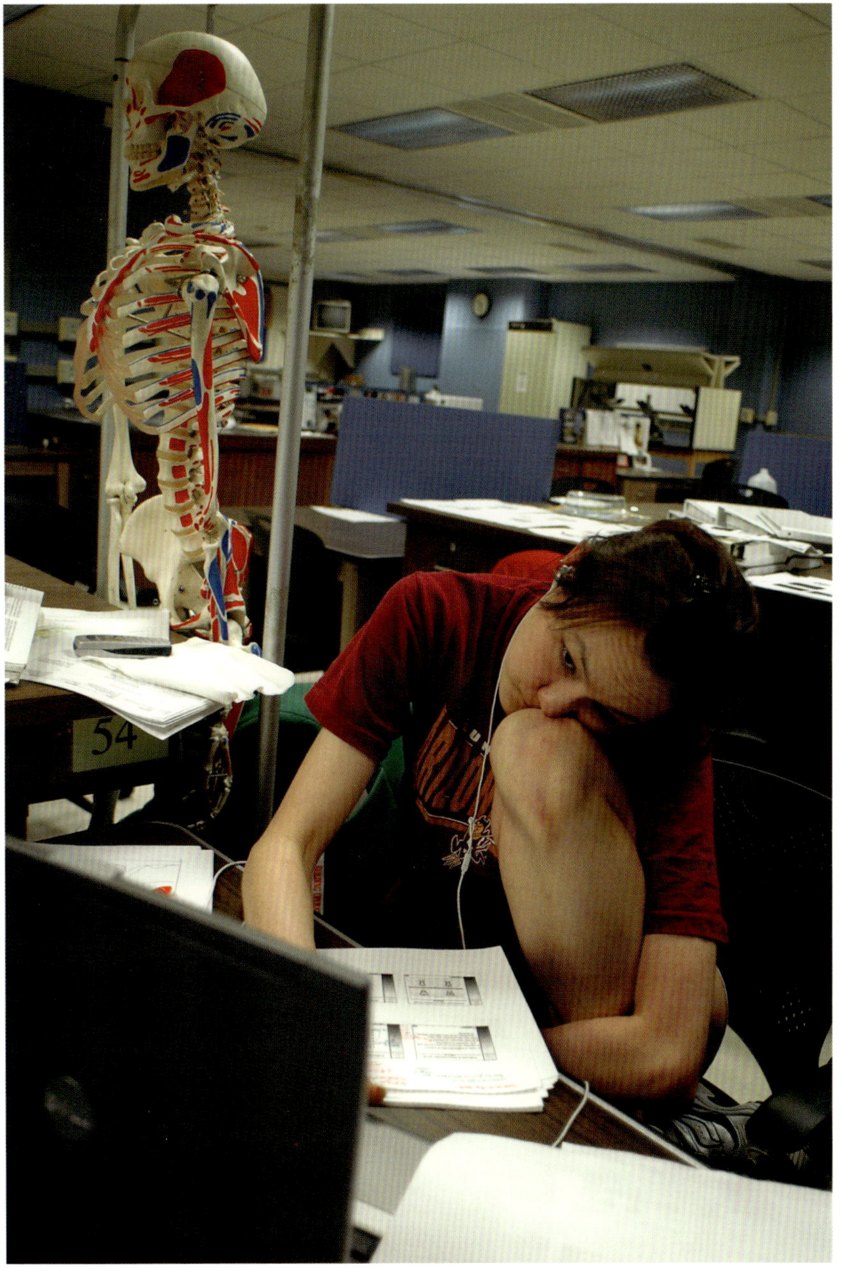

Sitting in a lecture-hall bubble for four hours a day pushed the limits of Gentry's mental endurance. She compiled shopping lists in her mind and counted wedding rings and bald spots. She started skipping classes more. She'd watch the lectures and transcribe them. This was time consuming, but she'd learned this technique. Writing everything down would make the material stick, she hoped. Some days, though, she didn't go to class or transcribe the lectures. She lay in bed wondering why she was there, why she'd chosen medicine. She'd always been good at science, always liked it, and she'd always liked people. Medicine seemed like a good fit. But now she felt as if she wasn't *in* school as much as she was defined *by* it. She was a med student. Take away that description, and who was she?

The weekend before a molecular biology exam in early October, Gentry broke out in hives. Doped up on Benadryl and unable to study, she got an extension. That week she fainted in the hallway after a small-group session. At a University Hospitals family clinic, she was told it was just a virus. But she was also dehydrated and run down. "I screw myself," she said a few days later over dim sum at Li Wah in Asia Plaza. "I should be studying all the time, and I don't."

She hadn't studied all week, and, she was about 150 pages behind in her reading. When I talked with Gentry, she was often like this: clearly frustrated with herself but unmotivated to change. She wondered if she'd picked the wrong medical school. Gentry had graduated from a small undergraduate college where students received a great deal of one-on-one attention, and she felt more isolated from the faculty at Case. There were so many different instructors that she didn't know who would be able to answer her questions. She also didn't think Case was as progressive as some other schools. Gentry

Gentry often studied alone during her first year of medical school.

wished that instead of just talking about the poor in class, students were made to go out and encounter them. She'd heard of similar courses at other medical schools where students learned about the medical needs of certain groups through firsthand experience, such as wearing blindfolds to experience blindness.

In many ways, Gentry is the stereotypical middle daughter—critical, stubborn, and frequently difficult. Interestingly, her namesake, Millicent Fenwick, also surprised and exasperated people. She was a pipe-smoking U.S. congresswoman in the late 1970s who inspired the character Lacey Davenport in the cartoon *Doonesbury.* Like Gentry, Fenwick was stunning. A Republican with white upswept hair and smart style, Fenwick supported abortion rights and fought for human rights and other social causes. In the foreword to the only biography ever written about her, former New Jersey governor Thomas H. Kean said she was "the only really ambitious seventy-year-old I've ever met." She came to politics late in life after working as an editor at *Vogue,* raising a family, and being inspired by the civil rights movements of the 1960s.

"She was smart politically and not above a trick or two to achieve her ends," Kean wrote. "Once when we were debating, she finished her comments and sat down. I rose to reply. About three minutes in, I had the sense nobody in the audience was paying attention to anything I was saying. I looked over at Millicent. She had taken out her pipe and was slowly filling it with tobacco. The entire audience was watching, waiting to see if she was actually going to light it. They weren't paying attention to anything I was saying. Millicent won that debate."

Gentry said her parents were impressed by Fenwick's style, not her politics. Gentry's mother was born in Taiwan, where she attended the country's most prestigious university before moving to

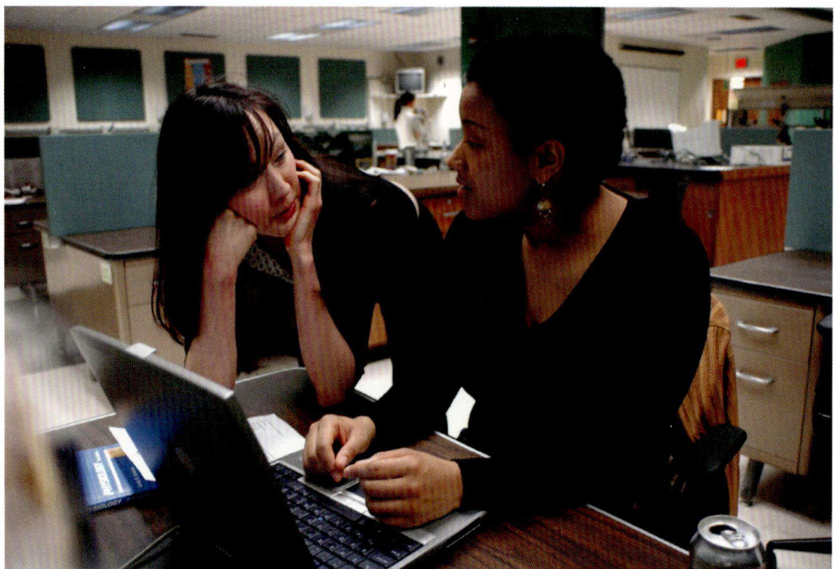

Gentry and Franco have a talk—and a laugh—near Franco's desk in the green room. The first-year students, like many of their peers, made second homes in the cube farms of the third floor. At night, especially before exams, you could catch students in the hallways and study areas. During the day, it was common to see students snoozing in the lecture hall or at their desks.

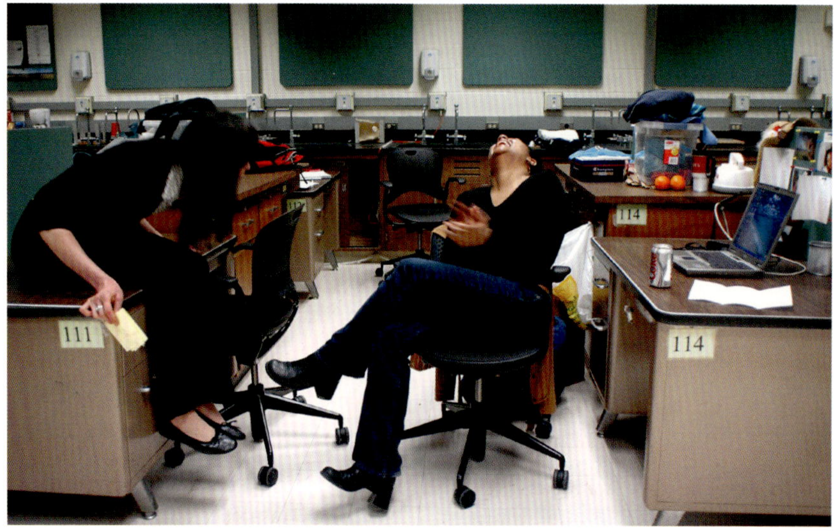

Alabama to sell textbooks. There she met Gentry's father, a former marine. They got married and moved to her father's hometown of Florence to run the grocery store. Gentry said her parents stressed self-sufficiency over everything. They worked long hours, and Gentry and her sisters learned to take care of themselves at an early age. Maybe for this reason, Gentry resisted the dependence she felt she was expected to have on medical school advisers, deans, and professors. She wanted to learn what she needed to learn to become a competent doctor, but she refused to "kiss up" to anyone.

Through November, Gentry continued to pursue a life outside medical school. On weekend nights, she went dancing at Spy Bar and enjoyed vodka sodas at the Boneyard, both popular downtown nightspots. She cooked. She shopped. She trained for a 10K. She skipped classes. She spent an entire day baking holiday cookies for her friends and putting them in their mailboxes at school. When she started feeling guilty about not studying enough, she thought about what doctors had told them about the importance of making time for themselves.

In early December, she failed the cardiology exam by two questions. For the first time, she felt like "the stupid girl." Granted, she'd only studied a little for that exam, one of four given on the same day. She focused her attention on the pulmonary exam and the anatomy practical instead. She didn't really study histology either, but she aced that test. She always did well in histology, the study of tissue. If she'd wanted to be a pathologist, she would have felt encouraged right then.

"I'm like the idiot savant of pathology," she told me one night over the phone. We were doing an interview while she tidied up her home, the first floor of a rented duplex. She said she had been cleaning all day and was feeling good about the immediate gratification of it. I asked, "Why not pathology?" She said she didn't want to search for disease in tissue samples. She liked kids, and she would consider pediatrics if she thought she could earn enough to support the standard of living she wanted and pay back all her school loans, which would total more than $224,000 when she graduated, not counting interest. But pediatricians were among the lowest-compensated doctors, earning between $150,000 and $170,000 on average, according to surveys. And they were on call a lot.

Gentry considered dermatology, which paid better and had better hours. It also happened to be one of the four most coveted fields in medicine, the "D" in the so-called ROAD, or lifestyle, specialties (the others being radiology, ophthalmology, and anesthesiology). *U.S. News and World Report* had recently noted that salaries for some of those specialties ranged from $250,000 to more than $600,000. Also, doctors in those specialties tended to have more time for themselves than other well-paid specialists, such as surgeons. But you have to be good. Really good, because residencies in dermatology are incredibly competitive. Failing a committee is a definite ROADblock. Toward the end of our lengthy conversation, after folding her sweaters and dusting her bedroom, she told me, "I still don't know how I'm going to be a doctor."

All three of the students said this to me at some point, but Gentry was the only one who said it with believability. I found myself reassuring her, though I knew I shouldn't. "Medical school is such a commitment," I told her. "You wouldn't have taken it on if you didn't want to be here." I felt a tug in my gut every time I said something like that. Unlike an anthropologist, for instance, a journalist's primary responsibility is to the readers of her work, not the subjects. If I followed traditional journalism ethical guidelines as I would if I were reporting on a Supreme Court decision, for instance, I'd be

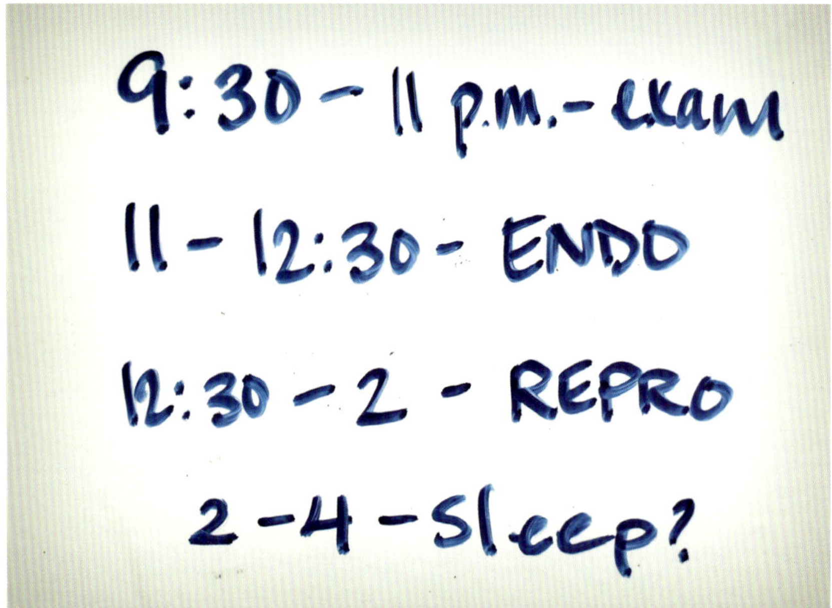

To study for one first-year exam, Franco planned to pull an all-nighter at the medical school. She scribbled this schedule for herself on the whiteboard of a study room.

little more than a recorder of what my subjects said and did. But I wanted the students to trust me. I followed them around, asked them questions, and rarely shared anything from my own life—the relationship is a one-way street in that respect—but my feelings were also clear. I did want them to succeed, and they knew that. But if they messed up, they knew I'd write about that too.

The cardiology instructors ended up throwing out two questions. Gentry barely passed the exam, but she passed it.

•◆◆•

The night before St. Patrick's Day 2006, Franco was planning to pull an all-nighter at the medical school. She wasn't alone in the green room, where her plot on the first-year cube farm was located. At 10:15 P.M., the lights were blazing and many of the small study rooms filled. Franco was in one of them, staring at her friend's laptop screen. Her hooded sweatshirt read, "Is there a doctor in the house?" on the back and "Case Med" on the front. She had written the night's study schedule on a dry-erase board in blue marker:

9:30–11 P.M. exam
11–12:30 endo
12:30–2 repro
2–4 sleep?
4–5 histo
5–6 anat
6–8 endo / repro

"So this is the adrenal gland?" Franco asked, dipping a plastic knife in her dinner—a nearly empty jar of peanut butter. Her study partner was snacking on dried fruit.

A student popped her head into the room. "We're going to do a practice test," she said. "Want to do one with us?"

"We'll be here awhile," Franco's partner replied.

In her cube in the blue room, Gentry was drinking ginger tea. Her hair still had streaks dyed red for a Fox 8 "Kickin' It with Kenny" spot she'd done earlier in the week. She was happy to be doing some modeling again. She even won a local competition and worked as a hair model for a local salon at some of its shows. But not all her distractions were nonmedical. She had recently decided to lead the Case chapter of the group Medical Students for Choice, a position she took so seriously that she even attended the national conference. In general, Gentry spent a lot of time in her carrel, where she kept a hot pot, instant oatmeal, and a variety of teas. If she had more discipline, she'd study first thing in the morning, she told me. That's

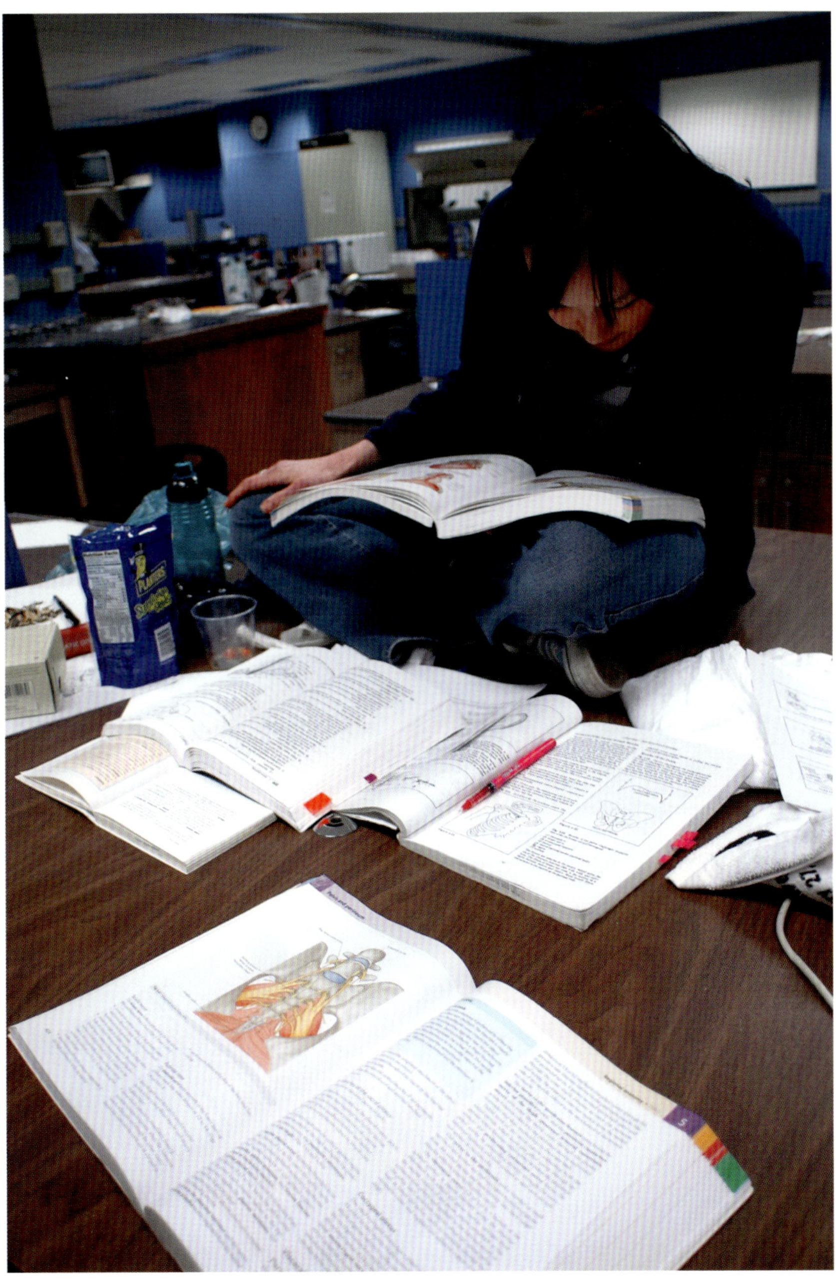

when she does her best work, but her more usual study hours are 11 P.M. to 4 A.M. After 4 A.M. is when you could often catch her walking home on Random Road. With the big endo-repro exam tomorrow, there was a good chance she wouldn't be walking home that night.

Franco was trying out a new studying strategy that mirrored her new confidence, courtesy of the mastery exam. Franco had built up the exam as the ultimate symbol of failure in her mind. When she realized she had to take it, she felt as if someone had emblazoned her white coat with a scarlet F. But she took the exam and she did even better than survive—she thought the extra studying solidified some biochemistry knowledge that would not have stuck if she had just squeaked by. She knew she couldn't learn everything. She no longer attempted to do so. She focused on studying what she thought was most important based on the professors' lectures and review sessions. She still studied a lot—five or six hours a day, sometimes with other students and sometimes alone in the law library, where she knew she wouldn't know anyone. She studied more efficiently, more confidently. She hoped that when she did need some medical information, she'd be able to access it quickly and act on it correctly. That, not complete genius-level retention, was all Franco hoped for now.

The idealist had become a realist. Ironically, lowering her expectations increased her competitiveness. When telling me about exams, she started throwing in the class averages, which she often committed to memory, and told me when she did better than average. "Are you a gunner now?" I asked. She said no, though she admitted to having developed gunner-like tendencies.

About one exam, she said, "I didn't need histo, but I decided I was going to rock it."

Gentry studies for an anatomy test on a weekday afternoon.

The Self

Michael Norton's wife was nearly seven months pregnant when they moved to Cleveland, and they had no health insurance. Back in Provo, Utah, they were insured through his employer. The Nortons could have bought the family medical plan Case offered. But at $3,244, it seemed expensive, and it wouldn't cover Kate's pregnancy, which was considered a preexisting condition. For only $910, they eventually bought the single-student plan just for Norton. Kate, who was unemployed, became eligible for Medicaid.

"Welfare mom" wasn't the sort of label Norton was comfortable with his wife assuming. Unlike many medical students, his family didn't come from money. His paternal grandfather, a war hero, fixed and installed air conditioners in Utah and supported a wife and nine kids on that paycheck. His dad grew up lower-middle class and worked three jobs to get through college. Norton grew up with more than his father had had. Bryan Norton was a computer programmer, and he provided a solidly middle-class lifestyle for four children. Still, with only one wage earner, the family lived on a tight budget. Norton didn't realize Ramen noodles come in more than the two flavors Costco carried (chicken and beef) until he was in college.

It wasn't until he was nineteen that Norton learned what real poverty is like. He went on the religious mission expected of Mormon men. His father did his mission in Mexico. Norton was sent to Brazil, where he spent most of his time with the poor and depended on the generosity of others. Norton wasn't allowed e-mails or visits with family, just two phone calls a year—at Christmas and on Mother's Day. Letters were his only connection to them. His father and mother both wrote him a letter each week, mailing them separately so he'd get twice as much mail. His father's letters—there were 104 in all—contained the contents of his soul, Norton said, "the gospel, [his] faith in Jesus, life and how to live a successful one. . . . They're a collection and distillation of everything he ever taught me."

Before his mission, while still in high school, Norton stopped taking Ritalin, the medication that helped control his ADHD. For years, it had lessened the nervous behaviors that others found annoying, including his habits of clicking his pen repeatedly and taking his watch on and off, on and off. But the drug had drawbacks. When he took it, he could focus, then thirteen to fourteen hours later—bam—he crashed. He wanted to stay off the medication while doing his mission. So in Brazil, he struggled with both distraction and poverty. Still, he learned Portuguese. He ate with other poor people, usually whatever they offered him when he visited. After two years, he returned home with a touchier stomach and a deeper compassion for the less fortunate.

Socially and politically, though, Norton was a conservative. He considered health care not a right but a privilege "I'm going to extend to everyone I can." He realized, of course, that it was getting harder to be that kind of doctor. Insurance companies were limiting options. Reimbursements to health-care providers were shrinking. Doctors had to squeeze in more patients, whom they had less time to see and get to know. He said that when he became a physician, a cardiologist perhaps, he would try to follow his conscience. But as a med student, he wasn't sure he wanted to be dependent on the state's generosity. He felt should be able to afford his wife's health care. Putting his wife on Medicaid was a huge blow to his pride, to his belief that only the poorest, most desperate people should ask for government handouts.

So much has been written about the intellectual, emotional, and cultural transformation students undergo in medical school. Scholars have studied aspects of it, particularly students' first encounters with cadavers, their tendencies toward depression, and their initiation into the medical culture. Students have chronicled their transformations themselves, privately in their journals and publicly in countless blogs and published memoirs. But there hasn't been much published by more objective sources on the sort of personal sacrifices people make to earn the doctorate of medicine. There are the obvious things: time and money. But what about the effects medical school has on self-esteem, on pride, on happiness?

There's a misconception that when you get into medical school, you're set. Provided you don't write bogus prescriptions for narcotics or accidently remove the wrong leg in surgery, doctors will always have well-paying jobs in America. Families take tremendous pride in children and grandchildren who earn the doctorate of medicine. I remember the hoopla when my cousin, who is now an orthopedic surgeon, graduated from medical school. My grandfather was a math teacher, but most other male relatives of his generation worked in the steel mills of Youngstown, Ohio. One of my uncles studied chemical engineering, the other became a pharmacist (and later a doctor of osteopathy), and my mother became a registered nurse. But it wasn't until one of the grandchildren graduated from medical school that my Italian American family wiped away the last ash-choked soil from its shoes. The MD was at the top of the professional hierarchy in my family, the sign that we had finally made it in America. When my grandmother was in her nineties, she always told people she had just met—people we brought to her home for the holidays, as well as store clerks and waitresses—about her grandchildren, usually mentioning "my grandson, the doctor," before the rest of us.

Unlike med students' debt and their knowledge, the personal costs of medical school cannot easily be quantified. Yet anyone who's known a doctor well has probably heard comments from him or her that directly address them: *I didn't want to have kids until I was out of medical school,* or, *I didn't want to get married before I knew where I was doing my residency.* They miss family gatherings and vacations, stop playing instruments and exercising, lose friends, and develop sleep disorders. And the list goes on.

I'm sure medical studies have always required some sacrifice on the part of the student, and I thought I would find some interesting stories in the university archives at Case. As of July 2009, those archives held 660 linear feet—that's about 1.3 million pages—of documentation related to the history of its medical school, but I found little about how students actually lived as they studied medicine in Cleveland. The archives can only be searched by provenance, the entity that originally held the documents, such as the Anatomy Department or the Medical Alumni Association. They cannot be searched by subject. The archives hold the personal papers of only one student, Zolton L. Klein, who graduated in 1936. They are mostly handwritten notes on yellowed paper. I found the most interesting student-life information in the school yearbooks and student publications. The yearbooks from the 1920s are heavy, gorgeously designed tomes one might display even more proudly than a diploma. Classes were small in those days. In 1925, there were only twenty-nine in the graduating class. The graduates looked serious in their photographs—and formal in suits and ties, and with oiled hair.

In 1852, Case (then Western Reserve College) became the second medical school in the country to graduate a female physician, Nancy Talbot Clarke, and it has trumpeted that fact over the years. However, there are few female faces in the yearbooks through the early decades of the twentieth century. The numbers improved in the 1960s, unsurprisingly, an interesting decade for other reasons, including the student push for more instruction in sexual health and disease.

In 1967, a letter from Peter Byers, a third-year student, announced a series of lectures and discussions on sex education for medical students. His class sponsored the series "in the hope that a program on sex education will be incorporated into the curriculum in the near future." The lectures and presenters included "Medical Students and Their Problems with Sex," by David Reed, PhD, associate in the Division of Family Study, Department of Psychiatry, University of Pennsylvania; "The Role and Responsibility of the Physician in Treatment of Sexual Problems," by S. Leon Israel, MD, professor of obstetrics and gynecology, University of Pennsylvania Medical School; and "Sexual Psychopathology and Deviation," by Wardell B. Pomeroy, PhD, psychotherapist, marriage counselor, and contributor to the Kinsey Reports. (Dr. Alfred C. Kinsey founded the Institute of Sex Research in 1947, one year before publishing *Sexual Behavior in the Human Male.* He and his team gathered around 18,000 sexual histories for his research, which was groundbreaking in the 1940s and 1950s.)

The last regularly published yearbook was from 1975. It featured plenty of casual pictures of long-haired professors, bellbottoms, plaid jackets, and dogs, as well as random sailboats and babies. There were a few odd pictures of students with cadavers and no captions to explain them. The last yearbook, published in 2000, looked more like college than med school, with many drinking photos.

The student publications fill only one box. The most interesting is *OB* (*Official Business, Inc.*), which was described in a 1971 issue as a student newsletter. "We will make an effort to print anything that any student submits, from far-out philosophy to kooky classifieds," the editor wrote. A new issue was placed in mailboxes every Monday. It looks as if *OB* was published for ten years, from 1970 to 1980. The first issues of *OB* are just copied and stapled sheets of letter-size paper, mostly announcements and other happenings of interest written in an informal tone. In the mid-1970s, the articles got more activist oriented, mirroring the social unrest of the times. *OB* published some railings against professors for misogynistic lectures and unfair exams. A writer for the February 16, 1976, issue explained why a lab exercise requiring the killing of a dog in cardiovascular physiology had little value for him. *The Interphase,* the student publication that succeeded *OB,* looks as if it was published between 1980 and 1982. Illustrations and cartoons accompany articles, poems, and other writings. The editors of a 1980 issue placed an essay from a physician trying to obtain Medicaid abortions for the poor above a handwritten recipe for pumpkin ice cream dessert.

The lasting impression I have from perusing the yearbooks and student publications is how accurately the students reflected their generations. There is a sense, even in the last yearbook, published just ten years ago, that med school is another world, and the yearbooks captured that world in scientific catalog fashion. They include names, black-and-white snapshots, and sometimes poems and

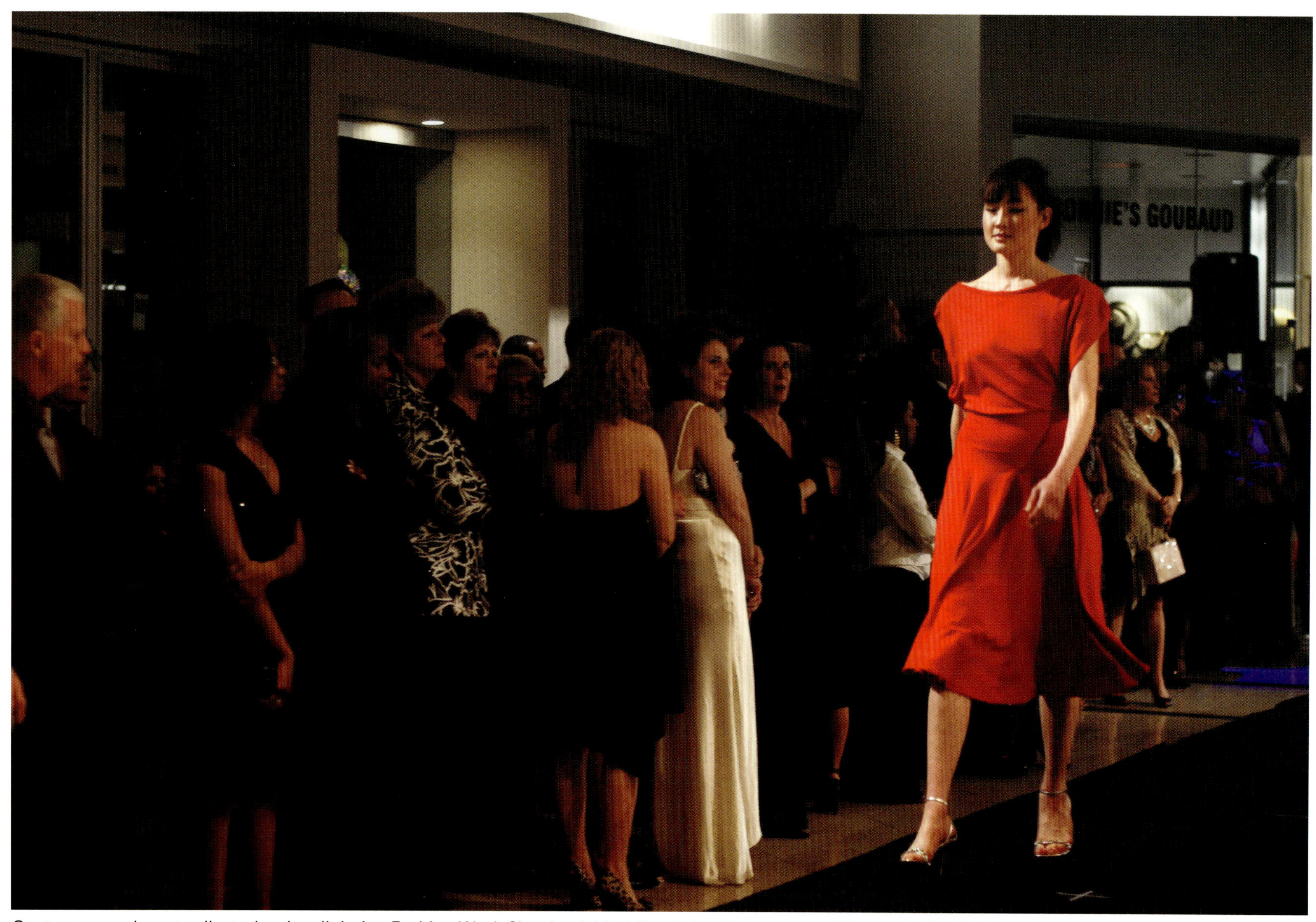

Gentry graces the catwalk at a local mall during Fashion Week Cleveland. Modeling helped her get out of the med-school bubble she desperately wanted to escape.

quotes. From the 1975 yearbook, a poem, "Frozen Sections from a Med Student's Diary," illustrated the exhaustion med students often feel in a comic light:

It's Saturday A.M. once more.
I stayed up 'til quarter past four
Attempting some rote
With each lecture note
'Til my syllabus caused me to snore.

The class of 2009 reflected the millennial generation (those born from about 1981 through 1992) in both dress—wearing flip-flops and T-shirts to clinic, why not?—and disposition. They were a casual-looking group, but also quite varied in their politics and preoccupations. They were on Facebook and Instant Messenger much of the day, mobile phones always turned on, laptops in their backpacks. Multitasking seemed natural to them, and despite all their schoolwork, many found time to volunteer at the local free clinic and get involved in other extracurricular activities, such as sports and school organizations. One extracurricular activity showcases the students' dedication to a cause, as well as their theatrical skills, more than the rest: Doc Opera, an annual variety show that raises money for charity. Student-orchestrated and uncensored, Doc Opera is song. It's dance. It's the one opportunity students get to relieve their stress by poking fun at the school, the profession, and themselves.

Inspired by sex, drugs, and rock 'n' roll—and a few show tunes, country ditties, and hip-hop rhymes—the 2006 Doc Opera was performed on March 25 at the Lakewood Civic Auditorium. Mary Poppins would not have approved of the song "Chlamygonnoherpesyphillexpialidocious," though the Blues Brothers probably would have enjoyed "Hole Man" as much as the gastroenterologists in the audience did. The documentary-style commercial for "CaseMed and CaseMed Apartments" ("Come. Stay. Live. Learn.") featured footage of med students sleeping in class. In "Free Pen," Dean Ralph Horwitz—that untiring steward of professionalism—shooed away pharmaceutical representatives waving airline tickets to the tune of Edgar Winter's "Free Ride":

Come on and take a free trip
Think of me when you write your script
Come on and take a free trip
Come on.

Gentry danced in the show to "Send Him to Psych," with musical inspiration provided by Billy Joel's "You May Be Right." Franco danced too in "Giving You Meds So You Don't Feel" (En Vogue's "Giving Him Something He Can Feel").

After the show, the cast, crew, and members of the faculty and administration, including Dean Horwitz, gathered at the Winking Lizard on Detroit Avenue. The top floor was jam-packed with students, some still wearing their costumes, including one in full Kiss regalia. Franco fielded several compliments on her short black outfit with fishnet stockings. The only noncostume-related compliment she got was "Your skit was funny," before someone handed her a Jell-O shot.

Doc Opera reminded the med students that they needed to have some fun too. Yet, even on stage, costumed and belting out tunes like Broadway wannabes, they were getting acculturated. To be in Doc Opera, you needed to be part of the med school club. The program had a glossary for the audience; by the end of their first year in medical school, the students knew enough medical terminology to write

Doc Opera lyrics for any musical genre. Much of the funny stuff was based on issues that matter, such as whether doctors should take gifts from the pharmaceutical industry—issues the students discussed in their training.

Along with the medicine and the culture, students learn about themselves in medical school. This is called "professional identity formation," according to medical educators. Educators say that in addition to developing the knowledge and skills necessary to practice medicine, students also need to develop (or strengthen) an important set of values—humanism, accountability, and diligence, among others. These values help them become better doctors for their patients, but they also help them become better at making choices in their own lives. Whether it's Norton's dilemma about whether to put his wife on welfare or Gentry's decision to lead Medical Students for Choice, the personal decisions they made in medical school offered peeks of the doctors they would become.

One course at Case focused on the personal challenges medical students face—the only one where the students talked about what it means to be a doctor. They met in small groups—the same small groups that first met three days before the White Coat Ceremony to write the "Oath of Professionalism." The discussions varied. Subjects included reforming health-care policy and the different perspectives on universal health care. The goal of the Science of Clinical Practice (SCP) class was to reinforce the qualities that can turn competent doctors into great ones, including empathy for all patients and a commitment to continuous self-improvement and lifelong learning. There was a heavy ethics emphasis here. Medical ethics, the code by which one conducts oneself professionally, is always a hot topic, and a person's ethics are rooted in his or her core values.

I don't know if it's possible to change a future physician's core values. But I did see students respond to the message that they shouldn't give up working on bettering themselves just because they're working on becoming doctors. They learned something I always heard as a new mother: you need to take care of yourself in order to take care of someone else. Because of the heavy self-help vibe, however, students mocked the sessions, calling them "Touchy-Feely Tuesdays." The class met at 8 A.M., and attendance was mandatory. All three of the students I followed complained about that. They wanted to use that time to study. Franco slept too late so many times that she had to meet with the instructor in charge of her group. He had called her "unprofessional" for being late in the past, and she expected a tongue-lashing at her meeting. She got a heart-to-heart instead. "Don't ever think you don't belong here," he told her.

All three students talked about one particular aspect of SCP: an assignment to improve their own lives in one important, measurable way. They had several months to do this. First, they had to come up with a plan. Then they had to collect and analyze the data. At the end of the course, they would report on their success or failure.

Franco tried to figure out what would make her go to the gym more. At the last session before winter break, her small group met at 8 A.M. in a cramped room with bookcases, a stepladder, and a mini-fridge. They didn't debate any intractable societal or medical problems. Unlike when the topic was the inequitable health-care system or the epidemic of medical mistakes or the drawbacks of prenatal testing, each student had to carry some of the conversational burden while the instructors, including Dr. Ted Parran, SCP's co-director and an associate professor of internal medicine, listened.

One student, who wanted to read more for class, studied whether getting more sleep helped her achieve that goal. Another tried to increase the amount of vegetables in his diet by keeping frozen vegetables in his freezer. Still another, concerned about his acne-prone skin, analyzed how certain activities affected it.

Franco put her entire presentation together the night before. Wearing glasses, khakis, and her "Is there a doctor in the house?" sweatshirt, Franco turned her computer around to face the group. She explained that her gym attendance had decreased from three to four times per week before medical school to two to three times per week in August to about once a week in September. She thought finding a gym buddy to play racquetball with might help her reverse the trend. She pointed to the graph she'd made on her computer screen. There were more trips with a buddy than alone, but she still wasn't up to her pre–medical school workout regimen. So she joined the intramural volleyball team, she said. The end.

One of the facilitators noted that her presentation was "all anecdotal." He mentioned something about needing "outcome measures." But before the facilitators dismissed the group, the true goal of "Touchy-Feely Tuesdays" was reinforced. It wasn't about busywork and guilt trips. It was about making future doctors want to live up to even higher standards than society has set for them.

"Rarely will you ever be assessed by anyone in medicine who knows more about yourself than you do," Parran said. "Patients won't be able to tell if you're good at all. They'll be able to tell if you're friendly, affable, available. But they won't be able to tell you if you're able. My chief of medicine can't tell if I'm worth a rat's you-know-what as an internist. Only I can tell."

The SCP experiment, though it was small and low on the students' list of priorities, revealed something I hadn't realized before about the education of medical students. At the same time they're supposed to be meeting the school's standards—filling their brains with biochemistry, for instance, and doing well on exams—they should be establishing even tougher standards of their own. Someone wouldn't always be grading them, or even watching them, as closely as in medical school. If they don't develop high personal standards of performance, their patients aren't the only ones who could suffer. At some point, today's medical students will be interns advising tomorrow's medical students, then residents checking interns, then attending physicians responsible for all the students, interns, and residents working under them. In all these roles, they won't just be doctors. They'll be teachers.

The Patient

On September 19, 2005, first-year students followed a retired internist through the Samuel Mather Pavilion in University Hospitals Case Medical Center, a confusing complex of interconnected hospitals and other medical facilities. Occasionally, a nurse hurried past them in the darkened halls, her soft-soled shoes padding on polished floors. The students were meeting after hours so they could pair off in patient rooms and work on taking pulses, blood pressures, and patient histories. But first, they crammed into a large room with too few chairs to learn the basics of the basics.

Students were still squeezing past one another and trying to find a place to sit when Dr. Seymour Lieberman asked them, "What's a pulse?"

No one answered. He didn't seem surprised.

As the Physical Diagnosis instructor, he had to make sure students knew more than how to use ubiquitous medical terms, such as "pulse," properly in conversation. He had to make sure they knew what those terms meant.

A pulse is a wave set off by the heart, he said. "You can feel the pulse in the area where the arteries are close to the skin." Students' hands moved quickly to wrists and necks. Norton, wearing a white dress shirt and a blue-and-gray tie, sat on a table because there were no available chairs. He put two fingers on his arm, feeling for the beat under his skin.

"You are very lucky the university has a course like this," Lieberman said in his somnolent voice. "Anatomy's good. Physiology's fine. But you really want to get your hands on the body."

Lieberman asked for a volunteer. He felt for the carotid pulse in the young man's neck, the brachial pulse in the crook of his elbow, and the femoral pulse in his groin. Lieberman told the students to always examine from right to left, "because that's the way I learned it." Also, they'd have a better chance of finding the pulse if they used three fingers instead of two. As Lieberman examined the volunteer, he peppered his monologue with medical terms—"exculpatory gap," "systolic blood pressure," "diastolic blood pressure"—each followed by "Do you know what that is?" The doctor was kind in both his tone and his manner, even grandfatherly with his white hair and his friendly clichés ("Let's take a pulse. This is as old as the hills."). He answered many of his own questions, never trying to make the students feel stupid. After teaching how to take a pulse, he moved onto his next subject: how to take a patient's blood pressure.

Norton had been in class since 8 A.M. He was tired, but not as tired as he expected to be once the baby came. After going on Medicaid three weeks earlier, Kate had finally gotten an appointment with an obstetrician. The Nortons were concerned because she was in her ninth month, and she had gone six weeks between checkups. Even though the doctor said everything was fine, Norton still worried. The first few weeks of medical school had turned him into a hypochondriac. The prenatal tests only catch so many abnormalities, and he knew there's always a risk a baby will be born with some kind of disorder. Plus, so many things could go wrong in a delivery. He worried about the kind of baby they'd have. They knew she'd be a girl. They knew her name—Megan. What they didn't know was if she'd be hyperactive, as Norton was as a child. The young parents worried that Baby Megan would keep them up the way Norton had kept up his mother with day-night confusion and, later, night terrors. He tried to keep his baby anticipation more on the excitement side, but the worries kept surfacing. At the moment, he was fighting to focus instead on the mundane stuff medical doctors need to master—pulses, blood pressures, and histories.

He went with classmate David Svec to a tiny room where one piece of artwork competed for wall space with a busted clock and a hand-sanitizer dispenser. Their fourth-year student instructor introduced herself as Katherine. Her ice-breaker question: "So did you get to the biochem party?" Svec had. Norton had not. Norton was the first to play doctor. He walked outside the room, knocked on the door, sat down, introduced himself, and asked what brought Svec to his office.

"Pain in my knee," Svec said.

"Describe the pain."

"I notice it when I'm running."

"Have you seen a doctor for it before? Have you taken anything for it before?"

"No."

"What kind of pain? Is it sharp? Is it in the skin? The bone?"

After about five minutes, Svec told Norton and Katherine that he really had experienced pain in his knee when he was younger. Norton questioned him more thoroughly than the doctor who'd actually treated him, he said. Katherine told them it's important to ask a lot of questions. As an aside, she mentioned she was going into child psychiatry.

"One psychiatrist tried to diagnose me with bipolar disorder," Norton blurted out. "I've got the manic, not the depression."

Svec and Katherine looked taken aback by the statement, and I wondered if Norton noticed. Kate was Norton's social barometer. She usually had to tell him when he was freezing out his audience, but she wasn't here to prevent this inappropriate disclosure.

After a long, awkward pause, Katherine started talking about blood pressures. The subject of Norton's misdiagnosis faded to the sound of blood pushing against arterial walls.

Norton had gone to Brigham Young University, where the majority of students are Mormon. During his first year at Case, he was still adjusting to being around so many people who didn't share—or even understand—his faith. Norton was disappointed that so many student-organized social events took place in bars or otherwise involved alcohol. (As a child he learned what beer smelled like because his recycling-minded father would pick up the cans littering his daily jogging route and bring them home.) According to the official website of the Mormon Church, the law of health or "the Word of Wisdom" (revealed to the prophet Joseph Smith in 1833) prohibits Mormons from drinking alcohol, coffee, and tea and from using tobacco and illegal drugs. Prescription drugs, like Norton's ADHD medication, are permitted as long as they are not abused.

I knew what his church disallowed, and I knew Mormons tend

to have big families and get negative press (the polygamist compounds, the teenage brides), but I didn't know much about the church itself. The first time Norton said, "LDS," I thought it was a medical acronym.

"LDS" stands for Latter-day Saints, of which there are more than 13 million worldwide. They are Christians. Unlike Catholics, like me, or Methodists or members of other sects of Christianity, however, they believe the teachings of Jesus's apostles were changed after they died. The result was a great "falling away" of the church from the earth. God then began to restore the church in 1820, through the prophet Joseph Smith. Unlike many modern religions, the Mormon Church advocates a particular lifestyle. They tithe generously, for instance. They also encourage large families. "Now and forever, what matters most is family," the church says on its website.

Norton is a family man. Whatever the topic, he finds someone with some connection to it in his family tree or his branching network of Mormon social contacts. He is proud to be his parents' son, his wife's husband, and his soon-to-be-born baby's father. What he needs to accomplish socially he will do not for himself, but for them.

Ten days after Norton learned to take a pulse, Kate went into labor. On a Thursday afternoon, September 29, 2005, she was admitted to University MacDonald Women's Hospital, right next to the medical school. She labored throughout the night and the next morning. Norton called me while I was still at work. I was thrilled that he wanted me to be one of the first people to meet his baby daughter. At that point, we had done only one long interview, but it was a good one. Clearly, some degree of trust had been established. I also suspected the Nortons did not want to keep this joyous experience all to themselves. Because Kate went into labor more than two weeks before her due date, none of their family would be able to get there from the West Coast. At least they had me. I finished the story I was editing as quickly as I could. I still had a few hours before I had to pick up my daughter, Stella, from her child-care center, and I hoped I could be there when Megan was born.

Ever since I had Stella on June 10, 2004, I've enjoyed being around expectant mothers. As I drove down Chester Avenue from my magazine's offices in Cleveland's Playhouse Square, I remembered my own labor, how I feared it so much, then how quickly it passed. As I drove to the hospital, I remembered the indescribable exuberance of giving birth, followed by feeling that aside from keeping my baby healthy and happy, nothing much mattered anymore.

Norton's baby's life would be so different from Stella's. Megan would be poor for her first few years, wearing hand-me-downs and eating groceries bought with food stamps. But she'd also be taken care of by her own mother 24–7, an option I did not have, with both my husband and me working in the low-paying journalism industry. My child was the first grandchild in my family and had an entire closet of new clothes. But I went back to work full time after nine weeks and struggled to find a quality day-care setting for her for months. Norton's daughter would probably have more siblings—he had told me of their intention to have a big family. At the time, I wasn't sure Stella would have even one. My husband and I debated whether we should have a second child, given our busy careers and financial circumstances.

This brings me back to why I'm a bit of a birth junkie. Childbirth is the great equalizer—and a far happier occasion than the other great equalizer, death. All children are on different trajectories predestined by their parents' backgrounds, beliefs, and circumstances, but in America they usually come into the world the same way. There is a doctor to welcome them out of the womb.

By the time I arrived at the hospital, around 1:30 P.M., Kate had been pushing for an hour. Norton came out of the room looking exhausted, his clothes rumpled and his hair flat. (He said he had forgotten the hair gel he uses to keep it spiky on top, and, even worse, his deodorant.) But his look was calm, his voice steady.

"We're close," he said with a slight smile.

I confessed my excitement for them. As he walked away, I told him how well he was holding up. He stopped and shot me a look of disbelief. "I'm scared to death," he said. Then he rushed back down the hallway.

The calmness on his face was a mask, a really good one. I could hardly believe he was the same person I had seen struggle with a blood-pressure gauge less than two weeks earlier, the socially challenged student deflecting his classmate's attention from a patient history with his own patient history. Already Norton emanated confidence without being able to feel it. I always thought doctors had to be trained to do that—to sublimate their own feelings so they can reassure worried patients and family members. But minutes before his baby's birth, Norton already had that composure.

He maintained it soon after she arrived, too. He came to get me in the waiting room just after 2 P.M. The nurse was still cleaning up the afterbirth, and I shouted my congratulations to Kate from behind the drawn curtain. Norton handed me the tightly swaddled baby, and I almost cried, peering into her red, squished little face. Beautiful Megan. She felt just like my daughter did moments after her birth—warm and perfect.

When Megan started to fuss, Norton took her back into his arms. He cradled her close then shifted from foot to foot to quiet her.

"Hush, Megan," he said. "Hush. Hush."

It took a while, but she did.

•◆◆•

In the first year, Case Med began having students see patients in clinical settings. First-year students used to have the option of following a woman through her pregnancy and delivery. But matching students with willing patients wasn't easy. Administrators decided to expose students to the entire life cycle, another feature of Case's ambitious new curriculum focused on merging the studies of medicine and public health. In the two-and-a-half-month-long rotating apprenticeships in medical practice (RAMP), students observed doctors working in labor and delivery, pediatrics, emergency medicine, mental health, adult medicine, and end-of-life care. After completing RAMP, each student visited the same clinical setting weekly. Ultimately, the class of 2009 would have more clinical experiences than any first-year class in the medical school's history, said Dr. Dan Wolpaw, chairman of the Clinical Curriculum Council. The apprenticeships were the first time patients would see the students in their white coats. But the educational quality of the sessions depended on the preceptor, the patients, and the students' luck.

On October 25, 2005, Marleny Franco's preceptor was Dr. Mark Feingold, a pediatrician at MetroHealth Medical Center. Feingold was understated and serious, but the pockets of his white coat were filled with fun. Along with a prescription pad and tongue depressors, he carried a kazoo and two rubber balls, good for distracting toddlers long enough to feel a tummy or look inside an ear.

The first patient Franco saw was a young mother wearing tight jeans, a sparkly top, and an expression far too sad for her seventeen-year-old face. She avoided eye contact, looking instead at the baby who squirmed in her arms and sucked at her mother's hand. Feingold sat at the computer in the corner of the room. He started the seven-week-old's checkup by typing notes. Occasionally, he turned around to question the mother and say something, such as "Your baby's old enough for shots." When he inquired about the baby's father, the girl began to cry silently. He stopped typing. The girl finally spoke: the baby's father was shot and killed in late May, she said, three months before her birth.

Franco worried she might start crying too. She knew nothing about this girl's past, only that she was poor and dark skinned. She was not even out of high school yet, and already her life was off the rails. Statistics suggested that both she and her baby would get subpar care throughout their lives. They'd be sicker than people with lighter skin and more money. They'd get into more accidents. They'd be exposed to more environmental hazards. They'd be more depressed. They'd be at greater risk for drug abuse, diabetes, cancer, violent crime, and premature death. Basically, they'd live worse lives, and that just made Franco angry.

Feingold handed the girl a paper towel so she could wipe away her tears.

When he asked, the girl told him she was OK. Really.

They started talking about the baby, her eating, her sleeping, her pooping.

"Hello," Feingold said to the infant as he took her from her mother. He checked out the rash on the baby's head. It's called cradle cap, a common skin condition that causes the scalp to flake or scale. He showed the rash to Franco before going back to typing patient notes. Then he swiveled around to face the girl again.

"I don't usually do this," he said. He told the girl he knew a little about what she was going through. His father died when he was three months old, and his mother had to work. It's really tough, he said, and it's OK if she needed some help. She could call him anytime. He assured her his answering service would deliver the message.

She nodded, then he turned around to type some more. She opened her mouth and a question tumbled out, very quietly: when her daughter cries, why doesn't she see tears?

Feingold didn't hear her. Franco repeated the question for the girl.

Yes, that's normal, he said. Babies that age don't have a lot of tears.

The girl looked relieved. When Feingold told her the baby was a bit heavier than average, she even smiled. Franco gave her a look that said, *You're doing a good job feeding her!*

After the baby's checkup, Franco followed Feingold to other appointments. She heard him give advice on everything from how to prevent diaper rash (apply Desitin cream) to how to keep jean snaps from irritating eczema (paint them with clear nail polish). He gave a free book to each child.

Franco soon went from observing patient appointments to participating in them as part of the community primary care preceptorship, the next clinical experience for the med students after RAMP. Her preceptor was Dr. Patricia Moore, a family doctor. At Moore's office, she learned how to do Pap smears and breast exams. She enjoyed teaching the patients to feel for tumor-like bumps in a gel-filled model breast. On the last day of the spring semester in May 2006, Franco brought fresh oatmeal-and-chocolate-chip cookies for the staff. She ended up interviewing so many patients that she didn't get nervous taking histories anymore, but Moore thought Franco's patient reports were lacking. She was too vague, hesitant. During a slow time, Franco consulted notes on a patient they'd already seen.

"A twenty-two-year-old African American woman reported with depression," Franco began. "Her symptoms were overeating, sleeping a lot. She was here to get her Depo shot that was late—"

Moore cut her off. "I really want the profile to come alive," she said. "Use descriptive adjectives."

"She had a flat affect," Franco continued. "Quiet, reserved."

"Give us a picture. We like to close our eyes and see her."

"A twenty-two-year-old single mom who was depressed and reserved."

Better, not perfect. The patient came to see Moore for a contraceptive shot. Franco asked her something general, and the woman said she was overeating and sleeping too much. Also, her boyfriend was moving out. Moore put the patient on Prozac. When she came back a few weeks later, the patient said she felt significantly better. Moore complimented Franco for her work with this patient, picking up on her depression and not seeing her only as "a late Depo."

Of the three students I followed through medical school, only Gentry used the word "hate" to describe her apprenticeship experiences. She didn't see much action. There was so little to do in labor and delivery, in fact, that she flipped through a baby-name book and even took a nap. She avoided writing her reflection papers for RAMP. They seemed like busywork. When she finally got to them, they were late. Not thinking that anyone would read them, she dashed them off quickly. Not long after that, her society dean and the apprenticeship coordinator scheduled a meeting with her.

The subject of the meeting: professionalism. There was no excuse for her reflections, which Gentry told me they described as "angry," "flippant," and "rude." They told her it was up to her to make the most of those RAMP sessions. Gentry apologized. "I agreed it was immature, and I should have been more diplomatic," she said. "But I felt I didn't learn anything from it, and I felt they should find doctors [to be preceptors] who really want to take us under their wing and help."

The lateness of her reports—not their content or tone—put her in the last group to get a preceptorship, the clinical setting that students visit weekly to get experience seeing patients. But that was not the only consequence. Gentry's lack of motivation was now documented.

The Cadaver

On the first day of anatomy lab, I opened the door, and the odor of enbalming fluid flooded the windowless hallway. It clung to my hair and my clothes, even my shoes. I kept blinking from the fumes and from what I saw.

Thirty-five cadavers lay on metal tables, encased in plastic. Some soaked in a reeking marinade of embalming fluid, a mixture of formaldehyde, alcohol, water, glycerin, and phenol. Although formaldehyde is blamed for the smell, phenol, which prevents mold growth, is the chemical that gets into natural fibers, the one you can't stop smelling long after you've left the lab.

Atlases are helpful in anatomy lab, but human guides—the surgical residents—are better. The residents looked only slightly older than the first-years, but it was easy to tell them apart: almost all the students wore white Tyvek coveralls to protect their skin and clothes. The residents didn't bother.

I joined the students surrounding the residents as they worked. The students stood on tiptoe, craning their necks, looking for the place where blade meets flesh. They took mental notes of where and how deeply to cut. They were explorers looking for sleek, shiny organs, tough ruddy muscles, tendons both stringy and strong, and secret places of significance only to doctors, such as the spot where the heartbeat can be heard through the back.

It is an experience both beautiful and strange, one body taking apart another. I felt awkward and thrilled at the same time. Not being part of the medical profession, I knew I didn't belong in the lab with the students, who had more than 2,000 years of tradition justifying their foray into the bodies of the dead. The people who willed their bodies to science didn't know a journalist would be hovering over them, notebook in hand, thinking of the best way to describe their spleens. Still, I had read enough about the role of dissection in medical education to know what an important event I was witnessing. I tried to think of it as a big show rather than a dissection. Backstage, I would be watching the actors—the students—doing the medical-training equivalent of tugging on costumes and putting on makeup. They were speeding toward Act 1. I tried to convince myself that I had to be there to document it.

Dissection has been part of medical training at least since the ancient Greeks considered animal cadavers valid substitutes for human ones. After 300 B.C., Herophilus, the father of anatomy, instituted human dissection at Alexandria's Mouseion, which functioned much like a university in ancient Egypt, attracting Euclid and Archimedes, among other leaders in mathematics and the sciences. Nearly 2,000 years later, in Renaissance Italy, dissections were done in outdoor venues and even churches to accommodate the crowds. Later, medical

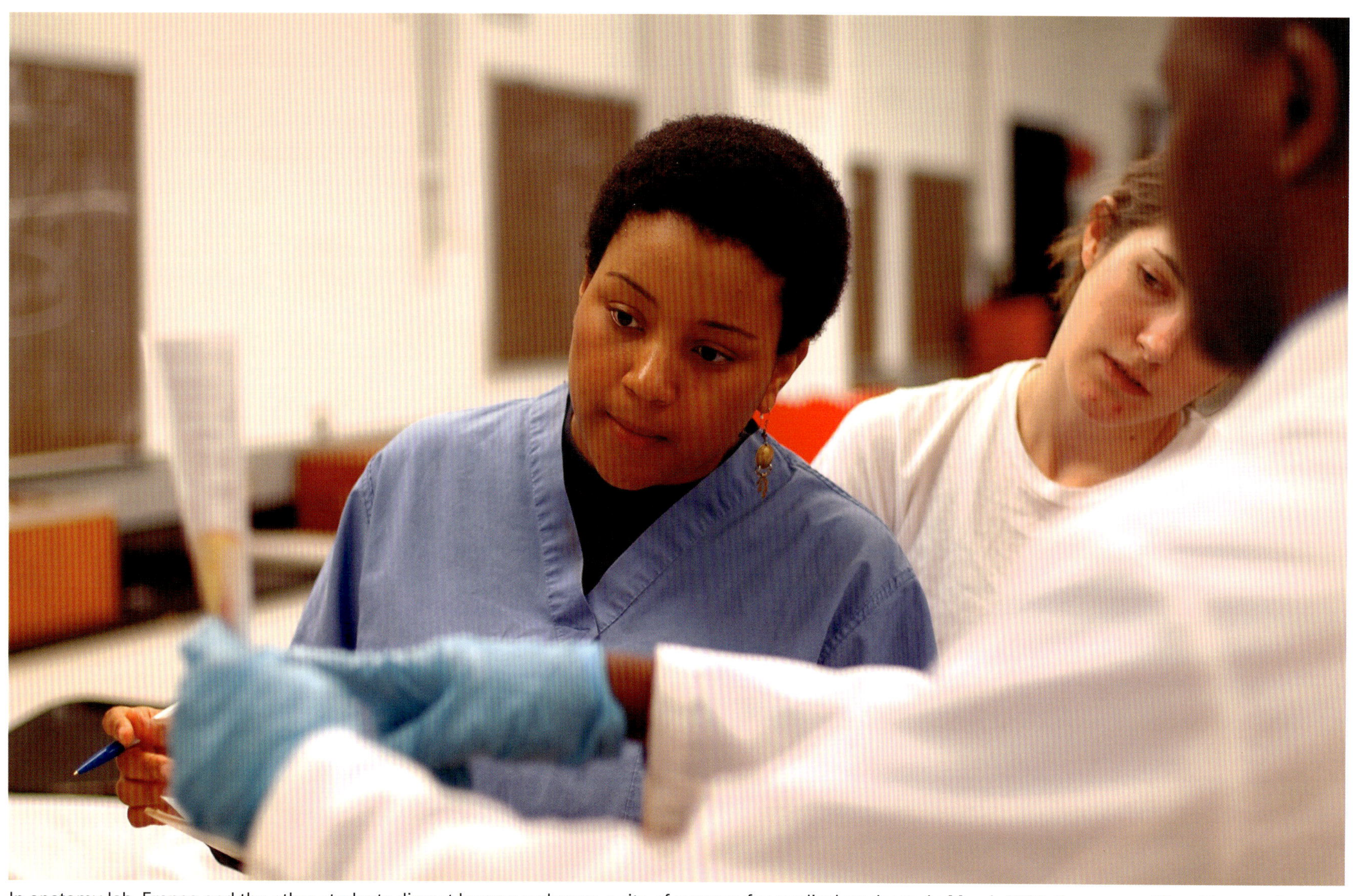

In anatomy lab, Franco and the other students dissect human cadavers, a rite of passage for medical students. In March 2006, they were still getting used to the language of anatomy. We often heard professors and surgical residents correcting the students' terminology.

dissections took place in anatomical theaters built specifically for that purpose. Some Eastern cultures eschewed dissection altogether. For centuries, religious barriers to the practice made it undoable in India, China, and Japan.

In seventeenth-century America, dissection took place whenever cadavers were legally available, typically after executions. Massachusetts allowed medical schools to dissect unclaimed bodies in 1831, leading the way for other states to do the same. But there simply weren't enough cadavers to go around. Even in the late nineteenth century, schools were still obtaining them through illegal means, such as grave robbery. Case's founders obviously supported this practice. You can tell by looking at the photographs of Western Reserve University's first medical building, which was built in 1845 on the corner of Erie and Federal streets in Cleveland. It included an "observatory," an octagonal domed cupola stretching twenty feet up from the middle of the roof. But, as Frederick Clayton Waite wrote in his centennial history, the proportions were not right for an observatory. The dome wasn't hinged, it didn't revolve, the rooftop underneath where it was built was not stable, and the university already had an observatory thirty miles away on its campus in Hudson. Many medical college buildings at the time had similar structures, and not because they expected their medical students to study astronomy in their spare time. The cupola was a good place to conceal cadavers when law enforcement officers were investigating a grave robbery.

"In its floor was a trap door reached by a ladder," Waite explained. "When an officer came to search he was detained in the office for a time. Meanwhile, the one or several cadavers on hand were taken to the attic and hoisted through the trap door by a block and tackle, the trap door was closed and the ladder hidden. The officer searching the attic found nothing and little suspected that over his head in the inaccessible cupola was the object of his search."

Because of spiking enrollment in Ohio medical colleges following the Civil War, the demand for bodies increased. Professional body snatchers, called "resurrectionists," were paid to supply them. Waite estimated that corpses were stolen from about 5,000 Ohio graves in the nineteenth century, wrote Linden R. Edwards, a former Ohio State University anatomy professor who interviewed Waite for an article in 1950.

Sometimes students, but more often instructors, secured bodies. In 1855, anatomy instructor Dr. Proctor Thayer and two students from Cleveland Medical College (as Western Reserve University's medical department was then called) got caught trying to steal a corpse—that of a poor person who'd died in the city infirmary—from Woodland Cemetery. The three were charged with "illegal disinterment of a human body for the purpose of dissection." The college faculty and trustees defended the instructor and students publicly, insisting the school needed cadavers in order to teach students. The defense was bold. At the time, people expressed outrage over grave robberies in the local newspapers and sometimes raided the schools. An article about this event, researched by the Dittrick Medical History Center, references "anatomy riots" at a competing medical school, Willoughby Medical College, in 1843 and Cleveland Homeopathic College in 1852. At the latter, the father of a woman whose body had been taken from its grave searched buildings of local medical schools. Even though he had no proof, he believed her body was at the homeopathic college and, "armed with an ax, he started for that institution accompanied by a howling, furious mob, which overpowered the police, forced an entrance into the building, and demolished its furnishings and equipment." Petitions supporting Thayer and his students, however, followed the Cleveland Medical College's defense of their actions. No violence ensued, and the charges were dismissed.

Finally, in 1881, it became legal for medical schools in Ohio to obtain cadavers for dissection. Over the past century, however, many medical educators have downplayed the importance of dissection, and students are spending less time doing it. In 1950, Western Reserve medical students spent 280 hours dissecting adult cadavers and those of stillborn infants in anatomy class, according to a 1980 book about the 1952 curriculum experiment by Greer Williams. In 2005, they spent 115 hours doing dissection. Many medical educators believe technology has lessened the need for sloppy, time-consuming dissection. With "prosection," dissections are often done for students. In addition to saving time, prosection allows students to compare the normal structures to abnormal ones at various stations around a lab. For instance, students can view a normal appendix in the cadaver, see a CAT scan of an inflamed appendix and do an appendix exam on a model or each other.

But gross anatomy committee chair Barbara Freeman said anatomy is a rite of passage for medical students, something that they expect to be a special, unrivaled experience in medicine. On the first day in the anatomy lab, "there is a hushed reverence," she told me, "and the anxiety is palpable."

Five days before the class of 2009 entered the anatomy lab, Freeman played them the song "Dem Bones" in the lecture hall.

The leg's bone connected to the knee bone
The knee bone's connected to the thigh bone
The thigh bone's connected to the hip bone
Now shake dem skeleton bones!

Freeman promised to put the song online to help them study. I quickly learned why she was one of the more popular faculty members. Funny, patient, and approachable, Freeman had done her job long enough to know what sorts of things to bring up before students had to ask—and student questions about a course like gross anatomy go beyond the basic what's-going-to-be-on-the-test stuff. What should they wear? Tyvek suits, gloves, and masks. Stay away from natural fibers. Wear glasses instead of contact lenses. (Advice I should have heeded myself.) What should they buy? The students would have a limitless supply of gloves and blades, and they don't have to buy the dissection kit in the bookstore. What if they cut themselves? They shouldn't worry about infection. She'd never gotten an infection from cutting herself in the lab, she told them, "and I'm 120 years old."

Franco took copious notes throughout Freeman's lecture, but many students just listened. Five days later, the students would be in groups, each group with its own cadaver, and the students wanted to know what they'd be expected to do with it, step-by-step. If they messed it up, they would not get another.

Freeman explained that they would be learning anatomy regionally, which wasn't the best way, but "the only way you can go about dissection and be done within the same year that you start." Limbs and back would be 32 percent of their grade; thorax, 22 percent; abdomen, 26 percent; pelvis and perineum, 16 percent; and vessels and nerves, 4 percent. She warned them not to blow off vessels and nerves just because it was last and it would count the least. Make lists, diagrams, and charts, she told them. Don't rely on rote memorization.

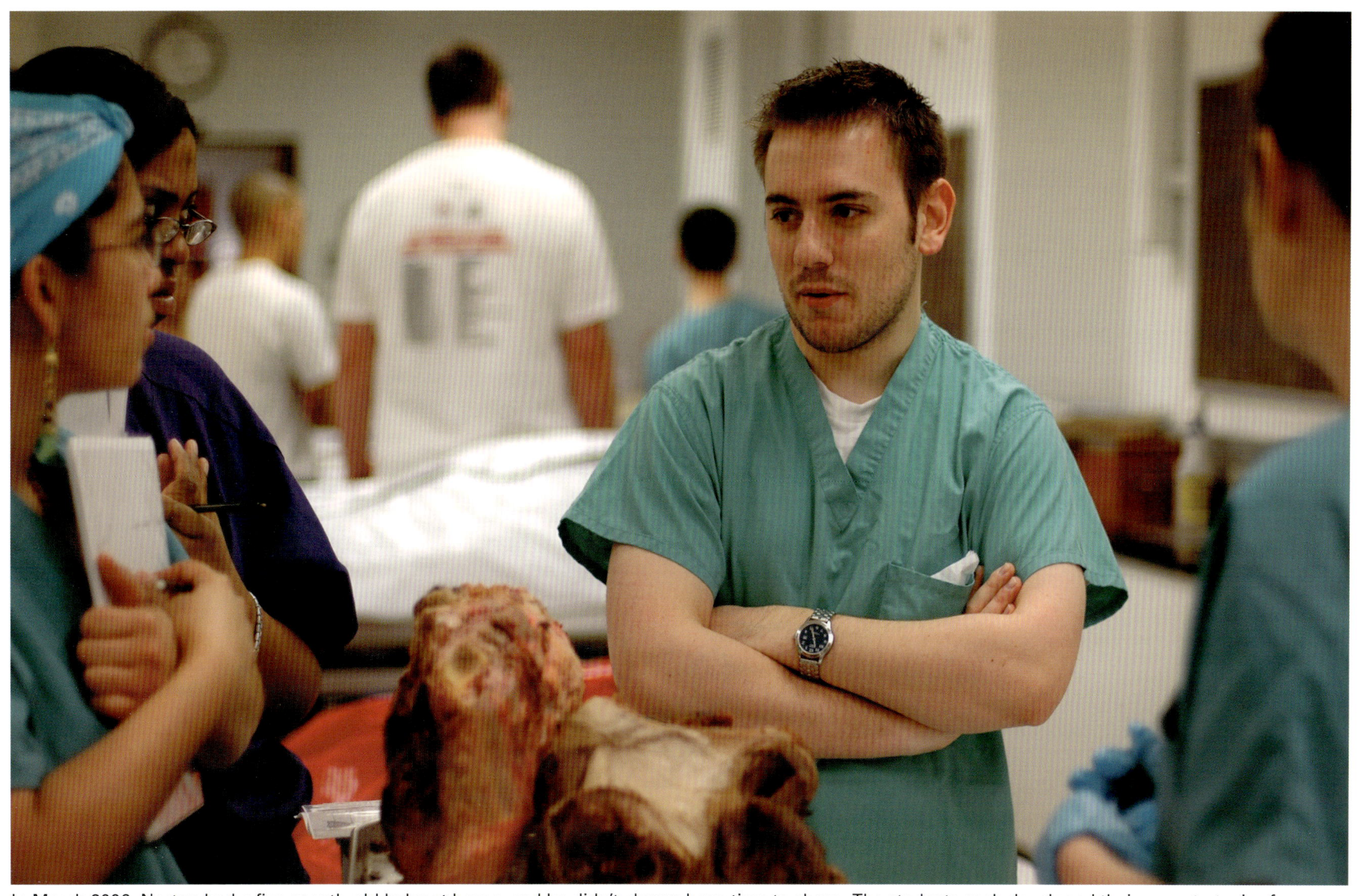

In March 2006, Norton had a five-month-old baby at home, and he didn't always have time to shave. The students each developed their own strategies for surviving gross anatomy. Norton studied images, but he found the information really stuck when he tried to explain it to someone else.

"Anatomy is not difficult, not rocket science," she said. "But never underestimate the volume of the terminology."

Freeman didn't talk about doing any emotional conditioning for the first day, though students do worry they might faint or throw up or have some other embarrassing reaction. Freeman had seen students faint and cry, but rarely. The first day of dissection is a test in itself. Can each student muster enough scientific detachment to slice into a human body, to take it apart piece by piece?

A year earlier, Norton had visited an anatomy lab at one of the medical schools where he interviewed. Even though he used to be squeamish—he hated needle sticks and couldn't bear to watch someone give blood—Norton didn't get queasy looking at cadavers in various states of dissection. He said the scene didn't bother him because of how he sees cadavers. "I don't see a person," he said. "I see a body, and the person is continuing elsewhere." Like some of the students Frederic W. Hafferty observed for his 1991 book, *Into the Valley: Death and the Socialization of Medical Students,* Norton viewed cadavers as specimens divorced from their human past. Students who did so had different anxieties about dissection than those who instead regarded the cadaver as a formerly living human being. Those in the biological specimen camp, in which Norton would belong, "were most often preoccupied with the possibility that their cadaver would look 'too human,' thereby causing them to falter from their desired detachment." The other group was more worried about losing a sense of respect for the cadaver, especially as the dissection progressed and it became less of a single entity and more a collection of pieces and parts.

Students don't just learn about the body they're dissecting. They also learn about themselves, about what kind of professional character they will achieve. "Professors counseled their students to cultivate gentleness as a counterbalance to the hardening influences of dissection," wrote John Harley Warner and James M. Edmonson in *Dissection: Photographs of a Rite of Passage in American Medicine 1880–1930.* That process has certainly changed with the times. *Dissection* includes dozens of gory but historically significant photographs, including pictures of students with cadavers and even postcards. "I'm awful busy," reads one postcard picturing a student who is dissecting what looks like a cadaver's jaw. "My tale will have to be short and snappy—Merry Christmas!"

For modern commentators, it's tempting to judge the students and instructors who took these photographs, to think they must have suffered from some character defect. But that would be a mistake, according to the authors. The proliferation of dissection photography from the advent of the medium to the 1930s, a time of growing professionalism in medicine, suggests that the photographers were driven by something besides macabre fascination.

The photos weren't candid shots. Some were class portraits taken with obvious pride in the dissection work the students had completed. Others showed medical students objectifying the cadaver, which was encouraged in order to obtain the detachment necessary to become a physician.

Hafferty's book discusses the oral-history equivalent of this: "cadaver stories," anecdotes similar to the cadaver postcards in their graphic nature and their attempts at humor. One involves leaving a cadaver's appendage in a public toilet. Another is about cooking a cadaver kidney for dinner. The stories could come to the students from professors, other medical students, or anyone else with knowledge of the anatomy lab. Hafferty groups the stories in five types: (1) those about medical students shocking nonmedical people with cadavers or cadaver parts, (2) those involving the mutilation or manipulation of the sexual organs of a cadaver, (3) stories about medical students "resurrecting" the cadaver and dressing it in the school colors or posing it to seem as if it had just sat up, (4) stories about the cadaver being someone a student knew, and (5) stories about the cadaver being used as food or a food receptacle.

Hafferty found that these stories, which were told as factual anecdotes, helped socialize medical students. "The activities described in cadaver stories reflect a triumphant victory over an adversary (the cadaver) who has caused them no small amount of emotional anxiety." The medical student protagonists in these stories have achieved the ultimate in emotional detachment, and medical students relaying the stories (or just listening to them) identified with those protagonists. Hafferty thought the stories helped condition medical students for the emotional challenges of anatomy lab and introduce them to medical norms.

The cadavers I saw at Case came only from people who donated their bodies for medical education. There were rules to prevent them from being used for any other purpose (including dark humor). In the many hours over many days I spent in the anatomy lab, I didn't see any cadaver pranks or hear any cadaver stories. I did see the students wrestling with how to think about the cadavers, about whether to call the cadaver "it" or "her" or "him." Should they see their cadavers as former humans or hunks of meat? They vacillated.

At least once per session, Franco thought about the life that once occupied her cadaver. Sometimes the hair sticking out from the plastic bag covering the head reminded Franco that blood once flowed through the body's flattened arteries and life once warmed its slack skin. Dissection of the head and neck happened during the second year, so students tended to keep the face covered till then. But Franco kept feeling a nearly overwhelming curiosity to look at it.

Emotional detachment came more easily to Gentry, who had been looking forward to dissection since beginning medical school. "It'll be like doing the meat counter," her grocery store–owner father told her. "You've been doing it for years."

The correct way to dissect, the students learned, is the way that allows them to find everything they're supposed to find during the practical part of the exam. Students worried they were going to cut something they shouldn't. So many of them wielded the scalpel cautiously, spending more time thinking about cutting than actually cutting.

Not Gentry.

Wearing an old T-shirt and workout sweats, her hair pulled back into a ponytail, Gentry made the first unhesitating slice into the tough muddy-brown skin of her group's cadaver, a man who'd died of cancer. She plunged her scalpel into the skin covering the occipital bone at the top of the neck then drew it down to the coccyx. Dislodging the skin on the back took a while. A few of her group members took turns cutting and snipping away at the fat coating the muscles. It was hard, messy work. The fumes made Gentry's eyes water, and other students' noses run. By the time she started slicing into the arm, her gloves had turned slick and slippery. Chunks of yellowish fat stuck to them.

One of the members of her group held up the arm as she carved into it. When she pulled a flap of back skin off and tucked it under the cadaver's arm, the muscles were visible, earth-colored striations with even more fat sticking to them.

Fat was everywhere. She looked up to see globs of it dripping off one student's glasses. On his way to a garbage can labeled "Human Tissue Only," he stopped to explain that the fat had splashed on his glasses as he was cutting. The other students took a long look. No one said, "Ewww."

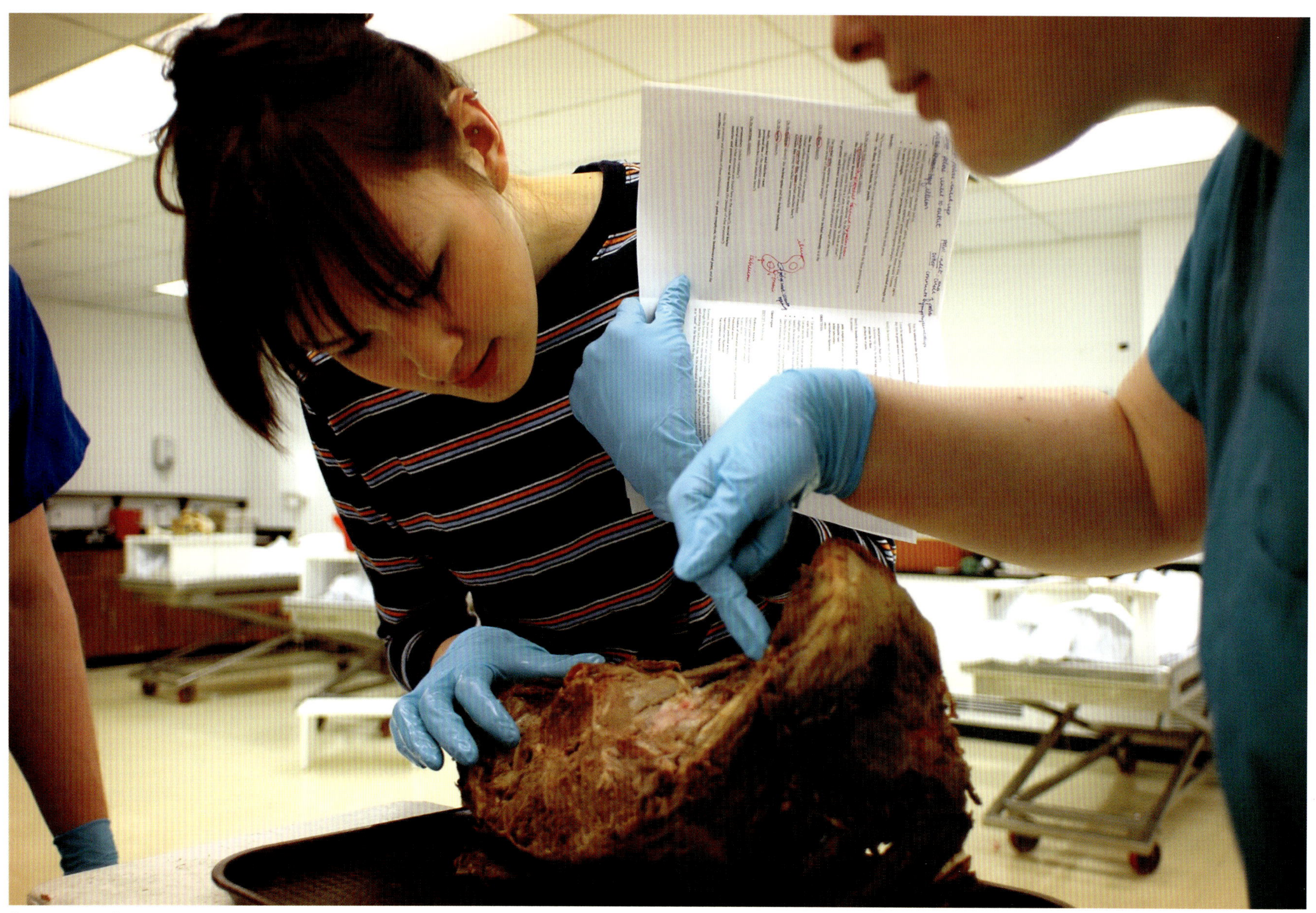
Gentry examines a prosected human pelvis during a tutoring session.

A resident told Gentry's group to be careful under the muscle because of all the blood vessels and nerves there. Gentry only knew the muscles she recognized from the illustrations on the Nautilus machine.

"It's going to be so much fun working out at the gym today," she said, smiling, finally in her element.

She wished medical school were more about *doing*. But so much of it so far had been thinking, memorizing, analyzing, and learning how to think, memorize, and analyze better. At the end of three hours standing, holding a scalpel and carving into the back, anatomy's novelty was already fading for her. Despite what Freeman had said at their introduction to anatomy, Gentry didn't see how she could get through the committee without spending huge amounts of time memorizing the terms. And soon it would be back to the lecture hall, where staying focused was so difficult.

During one lab, an anatomist joined Franco and Norton's group, sliding his hand under the trapezius muscle and lifting it to show them the rhomboid major and rhomboid minor. When Franco asked him something, using the word "upper," he cut her off.

"You need to use terms like 'superior,' 'inferior,' 'major,' and 'minor,' not 'upper' and 'lower,'" he said.

Like Freeman said, anatomy is a new language. If you want to learn it well, you need to do more than read and attend lectures and labs. Gentry drew pictures that she turned into stories, including one about the brachial plexus, a network of nerves in the armpit, featuring "dudes" and "girls." Norton learned by studying images. He found the material really stuck when he tried to teach it to someone else. Franco studied with upperclassmen. She also used flash cards and mnemonics. The students made some up themselves. Some were passed down. All were raunchy. "Steven Tyler likes sex and pot," for the branches of an artery, for instance. And for bones of the wrist: "Scared lovers try positions that they cannot handle." It was, in effect, an end-justifies-the-means sort of endeavor. How did they learn the anatomy? Any way they could.

The studying lasted into the early morning of exam day. Franco, wearing a sweatshirt and pajama bottoms, worked in groups and alone at her desk through the night, sleeping for just forty-five minutes on a couch on the fourth-floor lounge. Everyone was stressed. One student actually pulled out strands of her hair.

For the practical part of the exam, the students traveled from station to station in the lab, trying to identify structures tagged with colored flag pins. The cadavers, most on their stomachs and dissected in some places down to the bone, looked like real human pin cushions, pierced across their backs and arms. The joints were waxy and dull, like things a dog would enjoy chewing on. The limbs were elevated on blocks, the fingernails and toenails often long and jagged. Some still had polish on them.

In the lab, Norton seemed deflated in his green scrubs, as if the sharp tip of the pencil sticking out from behind his ear had just punctured his frame. Two days ago he'd woken up with a debilitating migraine, the kind where you see double images and colored spots. He was better yesterday. If this were college, he could just cram. But you can't cram anatomy. There is just too much to learn.

He hadn't followed the schedule he needed to keep it all manageable—and to keep his ADHD in check. His medication, Dexedrine, a stimulant, helped control the symptoms, but it wasn't ideal. He thought it caused his migraines. And he had to take the drug early in the morning because it made him stay awake for the next thirteen to fourteen hours. It made him really tired in the evening, often causing him to fall asleep while studying in the scoop-shaped chair in his bedroom. (After his nap, though, he could study for another eight hours.)

Routine was the answer. Routine in studying—reading before class, highlighting, underlining, and boxing important information. And routine in the rest of his life—cleaning, reading Scripture, having regular family time, every day. But since he'd become a father, routine had been as elusive as sleep with a six-week-old who drifted off only when she was held. To complicate things, Baby Megan had a cold. And Norton had just caught it.

A bell rang, and Norton, congested and miserable, moved to a cadaver with a pin sticking out of its chest. He bent down to study it. Then he scribbled the answer on his clipboard. "That one was easy," he whispered, relieved. Then he moved to a station with a pin sticking out of a thumb. Question: "What spinal segment supplies the skin pierced by the red flag pin?"

With exactly seventy-five seconds before the bell rang again, signaling a move to the next station, the look on his face was not so certain.

The cadaver on which he had to identify structures was the one his group was dissecting. It was the body of a ninety-four-year-old woman who'd died of multiple-organ failure. The cadaver was twisted, as if the woman had died just as she was trying to get up off of the floor. Norton walked out of the lab after visiting all twenty-five stations; he was sweating.

"Sixty-five percent is passing," he said. "If I blew it, then oh well. I'll just have to work harder."

A friend who was heading to the lab to take the practical exam with the next group passed him in the hall. "How'd it go?" he asked.

"What the hell, man," Norton said. After the friend passed, Nor-

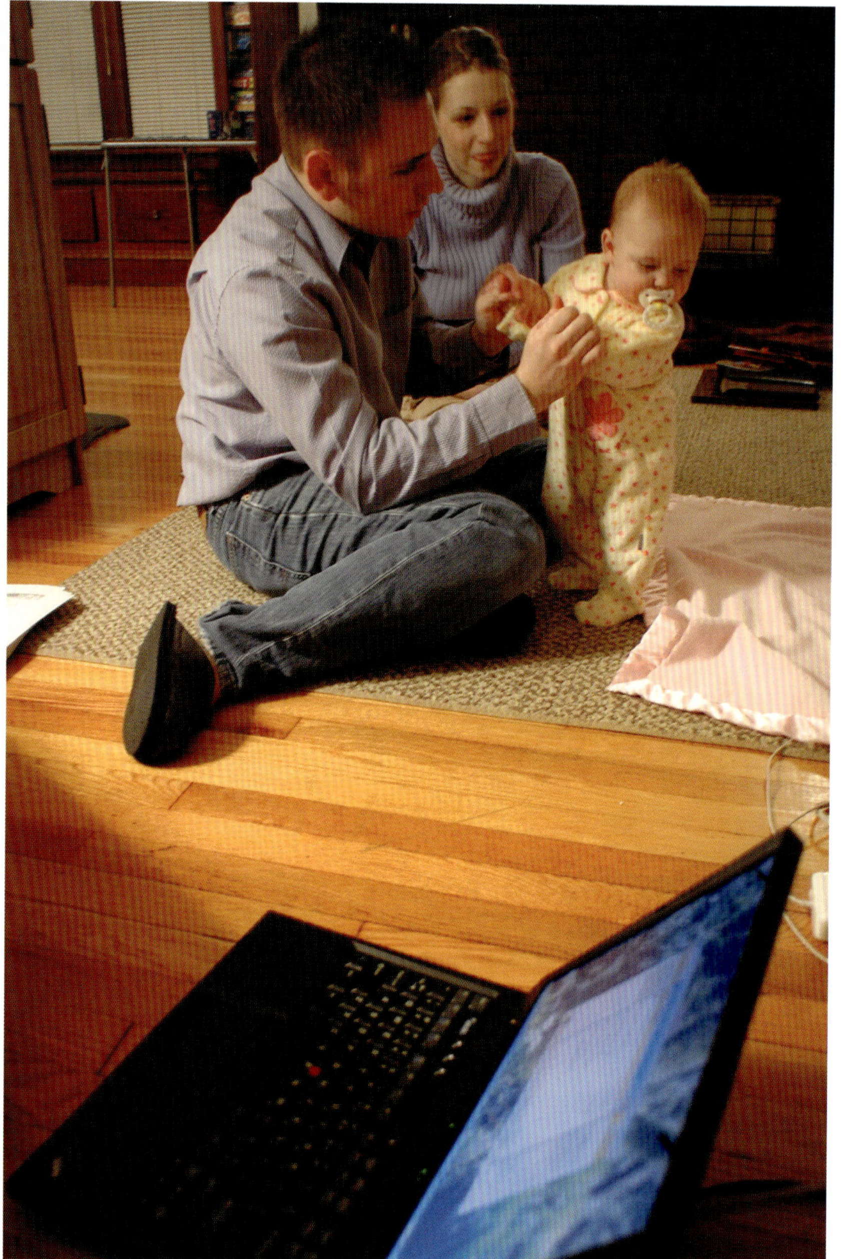

Norton takes a break from his studies to play with his baby daughter, Megan, before her bedtime. He did most of his studying at home, where he could be near his family.

ton added, "Sometimes, unless you spend 900 hours studying it, you're not going to know."

He worried he'd failed. And for someone who hadn't gotten a C since seventh grade, that was hard to take. He remembered how much that C disappointed his father. *You're not going to become a doctor if you keep getting C's,* the elder Norton told him. (That was the last C he ever got.) When he wasn't being exceptional, Norton felt he was letting everyone down—his wife, his parents, God, his teachers, all his future patients. Sometimes their expectations—or his perceptions of them—were harder to carry than the burden of ADHD, which he had shouldered since he was a child. At least he was used to that. But he wore his new white coat like a promise. *I'm up to the task,* it said. *I deserve to be here more than all the people who didn't get in because I did.*

Norton stayed in the mostly empty lecture hall until all the groups had taken the exam. Then he walked through the test with the committee chair, who went through the answers. Norton realized he hadn't done as poorly as he'd thought. Maybe he hadn't failed after all.

About a week later, he found out he passed. He always worried too much about exams. He'd stop that if he could. He just couldn't.

• ◆ ◆ ◆ •

Over time, the students' relationships to the cadavers changed.

Norton found himself increasingly desensitized. The first day, he'd felt "creepy" cutting into dead human flesh. A few weeks later, he reached in and separated the connective tissue with his fingers without thinking about it. Gentry sometimes rested a book on her cadaver's bag-encased head or leaned on him. Franco felt the pull of desensitization, too, and fought it.

"I'm surprised that I don't remember that she was human sometimes," she said. "I just think, I've got muscles to learn."

A few weeks into anatomy, while working in the lab with a third-year student, Franco thought she wanted to look at her cadaver's face. She had spent so much time wondering about the person who once occupied that body, she thought that seeing the face might make her cry. Better to find out now with an understanding third-year student than with a lab full of her classmates.

Franco asked the third-year student to pull up the bag covering the cadaver's head. When he did, Franco saw an old woman's face framed with hair that was both dark and gray. The pained expression surprised her. Weren't people supposed to look peaceful when they died? Franco ran her gloved fingers over the ashen cheeks, wondering if she had anyone who loved her and what her last days were like. Did she die alone? Could she even get out of bed?

As much as the face saddened Franco, it was the still lifelike hands that unsettled her. The fingers were curled, the skin still intact.

She had to work harder at this, she decided.

During cardiology, Franco went after the heart. Using an electric saw to cut through the ribs, she worked until the whole breast area could be lifted off like a lid. The smell of shorn human bone was distinct from that of the embalming fluid—organic and strong, like the way a chicken bone smells when it's chewed. Franco cut the heart out of its cavity and held it in her hand, thinking, *Oh, my God!*

She was not the only one.

"I'm holding a human heart," Norton said. "This is cool."

On heart-dissection day, the energy level, which had been waning, suddenly spiked. The students went about the dissection with thinly veiled amazement, taking turns holding the disembodied hearts, gingerly washing them off in the sink and comparing them.

"His heart is super-big," determined Gentry, blinking from either disbelief or the fumes or both. She needed two hands to hold it steady. Her cadaver's heart wasn't even the biggest in the room. There was something in the grocery store produce aisle to match the size of every one of the hearts. The largest, padded with fat, was nearly cabbage sized. Another looked as big as a cantaloupe. Franco and Norton's cadaver's heart resembled a small Thanksgiving gourd in shape, but even it had too much fat on it.

"This is bad diet," said the physical anthropologist helping them with the dissection. "You shouldn't have too much fat on the heart."

In late January 2006, the students wrapped up the gastrointestinal part of anatomy. After that, they had a six-week break to study the biological basis of disease. Then they studied the pelvis, and it was over. They had dissected an entire human body below the neck.

Emptied of nearly everything, the chests of the cadavers were just hollow cavities. Even for me, it was easy to tell the good dissections—the flaps of skin were neatly tucked back like candy wrappers, and you didn't have to look too hard to find things. I detected a sense of accomplishment on a relatively high plane and also admiration for those who had done the best dissections. The experience gap between them and those already wearing the long white coat had just gotten a little bit narrower.

"This is probably the best dissection I've seen," said one student while peering into the cadaver of Gentry's group. "Amazing" was the way another student described it.

"Tell my group that," said fellow student Tom Ladas, whose hands were the ones I most often saw in the cadaver. Gentry called him "SuperTom." She wrote "Tom + Anatomy Forever" inside a heart she drew on the chalkboard near their station.

He pointed out the adrenal glands and started to remove the cyst-riddled kidney. In addition to having lung cancer, the man had suffered from polycystic kidney disease.

"We have to chop it open, right?" another group member asked.

The answer was yes. The kidneys ended up with the other dissected organs the students keep in a bag on a cafeteria tray.

Then the subject turned to lunch.

The Preceptorship

In March 2006, Norton started getting more migraines. He had to miss classes, sometimes losing entire days to the pain. The stress had him eating junk food like he was in high school again.

He rarely found time to get on the exercise bike at Veale Center anymore and continued to gain weight—a total of thirty pounds over two years. When he took his own blood pressure, he was shocked to see it was slightly elevated. At about the same time, Norton was considering cardiology as a specialty, and he thought a future cardiologist in his mid-twenties should not be borderline hypertensive. Along with his study-intensive schedule and long days, he blamed his ADHD medication. His doctor agreed, and Norton started taking Wellbutrin, a drug commonly used for smoking cessation and depression, instead. Although it isn't indicated for use as an ADHD drug, Wellbutrin seemed to work—and Norton's blood pressure soon dropped into the normal range.

But while his health improved, he realized he needed to adjust his study habits. No matter how little sleep he used to get while he was on Dexedrine, he could count on the drug, a stimulant, to wake him up and allow him to study in the early morning hours while Kate and the baby slept. As a result, Norton didn't pay much attention to how much he slept. When I pressed him one day, he told me he got about ten hours over three days, with only two hours the previous night. The Wellbutrin wasn't a stimulant. It didn't have the same effect. Now he had to find time to sleep. He worried he wouldn't be able to keep up the progress he'd made. Norton received better grades than he expected on most of his exams. He thought his undergraduate training in the sciences helped, but he also worked each day, even on weekends, completing as much of the recommended reading as possible. A typical Sunday during the spring of his first year: wake up at 7:30 A.M., watch three lectures (stopping periodically to do the accompanying readings), go to church, watch four more lectures, do more reading, go to bed.

I tried to catch lectures and attend small groups whenever I could during the spring of 2006, the second half of the first year of medical school for the class of 2009. I often saw Norton there, wearing a tie and showing off his newest Megan screensaver. I never noticed him acting strangely, but he said he wasn't used to the Wellbutrin yet. He was tired. Even though Kate was the one who got Megan in the middle of the night, he'd still wake up. He kept trying new tricks to get the best work out of himself, to stay motivated. Sometimes he tried a little Pepsi or a nap. He listened to rock music as he studied—Pearl Jam, Tool, Better Than Ezra—but not on Sundays. He never listened to secular music on Sundays. He listened to the Mormon Tabernacle Choir instead. Sometimes he played the piano.

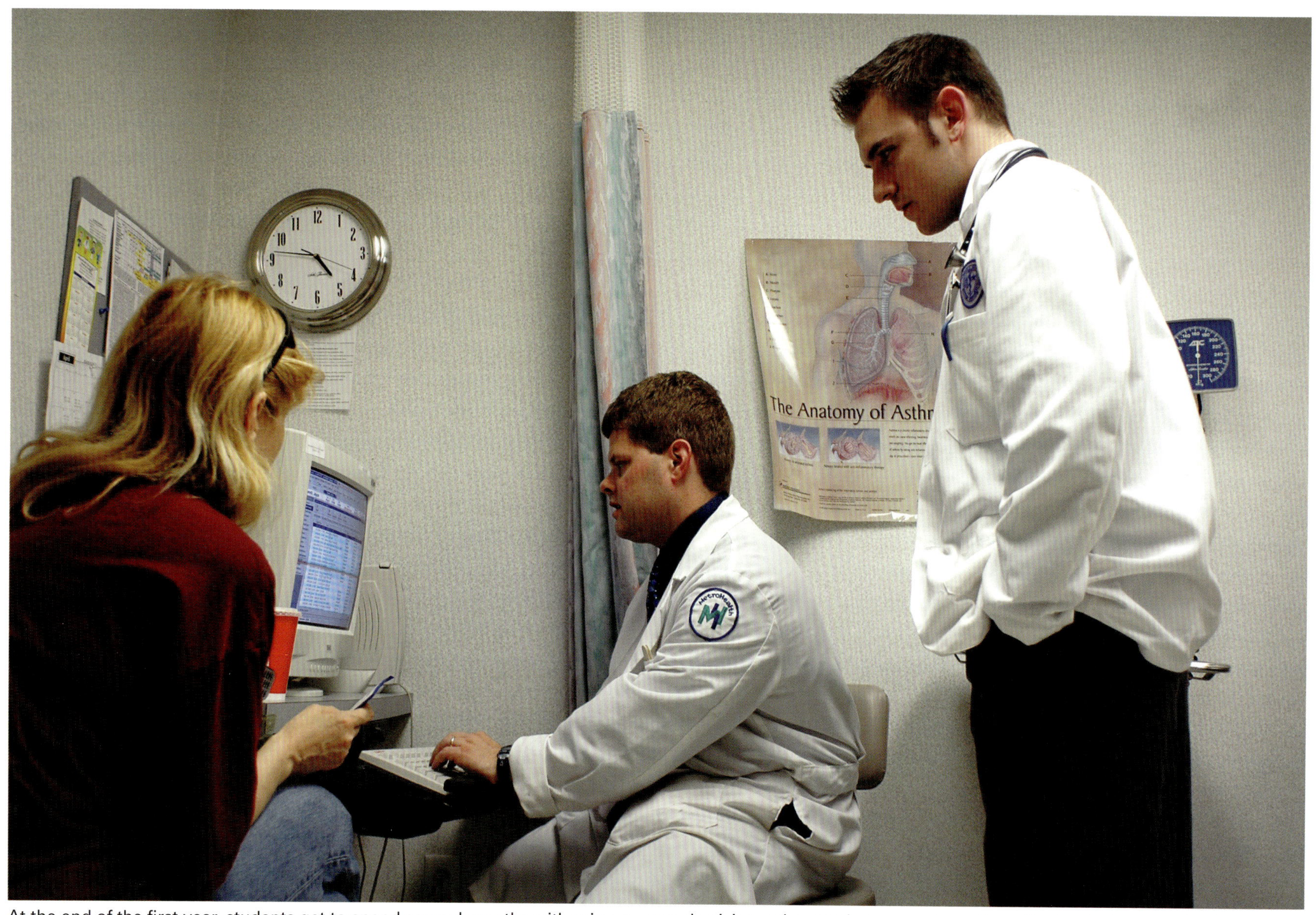

At the end of the first year, students get to spend several months with primary care physicians who acted as preceptors. Here, Norton looks on as Dr. Joseph Sage helps a patient in his Strongsville office.

Norton experimented with these study tactics as he began his community primary care preceptorship. The preceptorship exposed students to the gamut of conditions seen by primary care physicians. For three hours each Thursday afternoon, Norton drove to Dr. Joseph Sage's MetroHealth office in the traffic-choked Cleveland suburb of Strongsville, home of a popular mall and rib burn-off.

I met him there on a beautiful April afternoon. Patients were canceling—or just not coming to the doctor's office. That's because it was such a nice day, Norton hypothesized, and he wished he were busier. He wore his short white coat over a dark-blue dress shirt and gray patterned tie, waiting for patients in a sparsely furnished office near the treatment rooms. Sunlight beamed in through the windows, heating up a ball of rubber bands on the desk near where the Hippocratic Oath hung in a frame on the wall. We chatted about the Wellbutrin, about kids and weekend plans, in the unengaged manner of people expecting interruption.

Finally, Dr. Sage popped his head into the room. Showtime.

Norton walked into the patient room across the hall and introduced himself as "student doctor Norton." The patient was a woman in a hijab. She complained through a translator, her daughter, of back pain she'd had for six months. He asked her questions about the pain—where it was, when it appeared, its intensity. He took her blood pressure (which was high at 176 over 92) and listened to her lungs. He didn't tell her what she had or what to do about the pain. He didn't know.

Back pain is a common ailment. Treatments vary widely, from exercise to surgery. Norton excused himself and left the room to get Sage, who would know what to do. The doctor listened to Norton note the patient's chief concern about back pain and the absence of any identifiable cause. Sage made no predictions. They entered the patient's room together, where Sage retraced all of Norton's steps, taking the blood pressure (172 over 92 when he took it), listening to the lungs, asking even more questions. Then he turned to Norton. "Do you know what this sounds like?"

"No," Norton confessed.

"It sounds like sciatica," Sage replied. "Deep, gluteal pain that radiates down the leg."

Sage told the patient's daughter to tell the woman the most important thing she could do for her back pain was stay active. More than her back, her blood pressure concerned him. He suggested an increase in her medication.

The other patient visits progressed in a similar fashion. Norton went in first, questioned, examined, rehearsed, and presented to Sage. Then Sage entered the room with Norton, did his own examination, delivered the diagnosis, ordered the tests, and made referrals, while Norton observed and logged it all in his memory, hoping it would stick there along with the useless trivia he retained, including the heights of all the members of Metallica and random historical facts about World War I.

Together, Norton and Sage saw a forty-three-year-old woman with heavy vaginal bleeding. Sage had her lie on the table. He rolled his fingertips along her abdomen. "I'm horrible at feeling livers right now," Norton said, recalling a former drug addict whose cirrhotic liver he'd probed back in December. The poor man kept saying, "Ow, ow, ow."

"Start low," Sage instructed. "You can feel liver here."

When Norton did it, the patient didn't say, "Ow," once, but then this patient didn't have a painful cirrhotic liver either. It could also be that practicing on his wife was finally paying off.

In Sage's Strongsville office, Norton expected to see a mix of men, women, and children experiencing a variety of medical problems common to the northeast Ohio suburban population in the spring: sinus infections, allergies, asthma, bee stings, strep throat. What he saw in addition to severe back pain was incessant menstrual bleeding, a persistent cough, and chronic urinary tract infections. All his patients were middle-aged women. In Sage's office, Norton began to develop a definition of Horwitz's concept of "professionalism" in his own mind. Here, patients saw him in his white coat and automatically trusted him with information about their eating disorders, sexual behaviors, and mental health problems. They saw him as someone who could help them get better. And he felt driven to live up to their expectations of him. There were no textbook cases. Their illnesses were not isolated problems he could just eliminate swiftly and easily, Whac-A-Mole style. All required special considerations.

The patient with back pain didn't speak English, requiring communication through a translator. The woman with the persistent cough wore a shirt with the word "Sinner" on the front and a crucifix around her neck—Norton noticed this right away. She admitted to smoking a half a pack of cigarettes a day, a habit she'd had since she was fifteen. Her problem was probably linked to her behavior, but she didn't want to commit to quitting smoking. She just wanted the doctor to make her better. Another woman reported having frequent urinary tract infections since the birth of her daughter nine years ago. For nine years, doctors had just treated the symptoms, which went away with antibiotics. No one before Sage had referred her to a urogynecologist, who would be best qualified to identify what was causing the problem.

As well as Norton did on med school exams, he felt he was getting more out of spending time with physicians one-on-one, seeing living patients instead of answering questions carefully composed by medical educators. The roots of medical education, in fact, are in one-on-one instruction. In medieval Europe, medicine was considered a craft, specialized training in medicine. In the American colonies, the training was shortened to three years, and the "master" became a "preceptor," and the "apprentice" the "student." In 1840, Waite wrote, the student or the student's parents paid the preceptor one hundred dollars a year. He might live with the preceptor's family or nearby. He took no vacations. His instruction consisted of reading textbooks and performing daily recitations. He did animal or (when possible) surreptitious human dissection in a hayloft or some other private space when a body could be obtained. The student also learned how to prepare medications. "He ground the crude drugs with mortar and pestle, prepared tinctures, measured dosages, made pills, and became skilled in the technique of wrapping 'powders,'" Waite wrote. Later in his training, the student assisted the preceptor in patient exams, "learning how to open abscesses, dress wounds, bandage fractures, extract teeth, and let blood." His patients were almost always men or children. Students weren't allowed to take care of sick adolescent girls or women. They couldn't even deliver babies—or witness births—until they became physicians.

As the population of the American colonial cities grew, they attracted physicians educated in European universities, which provided better training. Americans who wanted a better medical education traveled to Europe. From the beginning of medical instruction in American colleges until about 1880, medical education consisted of two parts: instruction under a preceptor and instruction under a medical faculty. The first medical schools in the United States existed under the auspices of colleges of arts, where the conflict between lecture-type study and clinical experiences grew. College educators wanted medical students to focus on the science over the practical, and physicians—many of whom had come up through the preceptorial system—saw more value in preceptor-led education.

While the curricula of modern medical schools encompass both kinds of instruction, the students I followed at Case Med seemed frustrated that they weren't more intertwined. They wanted to think that the science they learned would directly relate to the clinical experiences they had. Too often, though, they felt as if what they learned in lectures and small groups was soon forgotten. What they saw in clinic stuck with them more. They would often start telling me about a particular clinical experience by rating the preceptor. So-and-so was a good preceptor or a bad preceptor: he had no time for me, she let me do this procedure or watched as I did that one, he made me feel like an idiot, and so forth. They checked their evaluations online as soon as they got them, eager to read the comments when they knew they'd be good. The not-so-good ones gnawed at them far more than a lackluster exam grade. In medical school, the preceptor, not the lecturer, seemed to be the real steward of learning.

•◆◆•

The second year of med school began in fall 2006. Franco took up salsa dancing and lobbied her father for money for a car. Getting around Cleveland by public transportation was tougher than getting around Boston, where she'd never even tried to get a driver's license. She bummed rides, and she was late a lot.

Even though it was often hard for her to get to local hospitals, she liked spending more time in clinical settings. She enjoyed talking to the patients—maybe too much. She made three patients cry before she even touched them. One was a sixty-year-old 330-pound former Air Force cook who came to the Louis Stokes Cleveland VA Medical Center for shortness of breath. He was in a partially reclined bed in a patient room he shared with another man, who lay flat on his back like a corpse, eyes closed, hands folded across his stomach. Both wore canary-yellow patient pajamas. The top of the ex-cook's pajamas didn't cover his belly. Grungy, frayed white socks with holes in them strained over his swollen feet. His nails were too long. There was white stubble on his face.

Franco had new bronze highlights in her hair and a well-worn copy of *Maxwell's Quick Medical Reference* in her pocket. She sat down on a chair next to the ex-cook's bed, took out a small white notebook, and began asking him questions about his family. He said he was the oldest of twelve. He had one sister with lupus, another sister with heart problems, and a brother with heart problems. Another brother died of a brain tumor at thirty-two. His mother had undergone several bypass surgeries when she was alive, but he didn't know about his father. He hadn't seen his father since he was seven.

"So your mom raised you all alone?" Franco asked.

It wasn't a question that would lead to any pertinent medical or social information, but it was a human thing to say, a gesture of empathy. Traditionally, medical students were taught to distance themselves from their patients. But recent research shows that empathetic doctors are better doctors, and Case was among the institutions trying to infuse its curriculum with greater humanity. Franco's class had been talking about empathy since the first day.

Until that question about his mother, Franco's patient had been smiling, somehow, despite all his medical conditions, which included chronic obstructive pulmonary disease, congestive heart failure, type 2 diabetes, glaucoma, cataracts, and erectile dysfunction. But her question led him to tell her about the daughters he had left when they were five and three. Through tears behind thick bifocals, he said he had written to them, and he was trying to get better so he could see them this year.

Although he could no longer do so many things—including lie flat on his back (it was uncomfortable), eat his favorite food (pizza isn't a healthy choice for people with diabetes), and have sex (his chest squeezed up too much)—he could look forward to seeing his daughters again. That dream kept him going, and Franco honed in on it. She encouraged him to keep losing weight and reassured him that his daughters were lucky to have a father, even a father who wasn't around while they were growing up.

She hadn't written a word in her notebook since his voice hoarsened with emotion. She just listened, eyes locked on his. After a while, she took out her penlight and shined it on the moles of his neck, searching for abnormalities. She pushed her plum stethoscope—a present from her mentor, Bob—deep into the fat on his chest, then into the fat on his belly. She lifted his arms and felt underneath them. She asked him to pop out his dentures and checked his palate.

Franco spent two hours with the ex-cook, asking him questions and examining his entire body, from the skin folds of his neck to the small joints of his feet. This was far more time than she would get to spend with patients on her third-year rotation, when students see most patients for no longer than fifteen or twenty minutes.

Having the luxury of time was both a tease and a thought-provoker. She knew she shouldn't get used to it. But what if she could? How much better care could be delivered if doctors had time to get to know their patients? How much better would patients feel about them? In medical school, there's never enough time for studying. In medicine, there's never enough time for patients.

•◆◆•

In medical school, whatever you know, whatever you decide, whatever you do—someone's always watching, listening, and taking mental notes or written ones. By year 2, Gentry's knowledge and skills had been tested in labs and on computer-based exams. She had been videotaped taking patient histories and performing physical exams. The process was meant to give students practice, but Gentry couldn't get over how fake it felt to examine actors pretending to be patients.

It slowed her down thinking about what they were going to say next to throw her off. One time she had a practice patient who was acting like a depressed fifty-five-year-old man. She got so nervous during the interview that she forgot just about everything about him except for the chief complaint then tried to make up for it by asking lots of questions, including whether he'd had a colonoscopy and a prostate exam. She was thrilled when the preceptor praised her for asking health-maintenance questions.

After watching the video of herself interviewing the patient, she completed a self-evaluation form. "I don't feel that I have a talent for interviewing patients," she wrote. "I feel that I could interview in a more organized manner. I have a tendency to abruptly change the subject and I feel that this might confuse and irritate my patients. I also feel that I could take a better past medical history, family history, and review of symptoms. I also feel that I could speak more clearly and with more confidence." She noted that she did treat the patient with respect, listened, and responded appropriately, but the rest of her comments were quite critical and specific. For example, she would work on avoiding saying, "Umm," and "Like," and maintaining better eye contact and posture.

After blowing off her RAMP reflection essays during the first year, Gentry was chastened. Still angry and disaffected, but chastened. All her life she'd been bucking people's expectations. Because she's social, people assume she's not smart. But she'd gotten what she deserved in medical school, so far. She'd gotten what she'd put into it, she told me.

She finally got a preceptorship at the Douglas Moore Health Center at University Hospitals Case Medical Center, where she spent her Monday afternoons. The center was located on the third floor of Bolwell Hospital, but for most of her preceptorship Gentry turned the wrong way out of the stairwell and ended up at dermatology. That was only the beginning of the bewilderment she felt at Douglas Moore. She often had no answers to the questions she was asked. She had to work through bouts of paralysis when she was told to auscultate (listen), percuss (strike), or palpate (touch). She neglected to ask pertinent questions while taking histories. Once she forgot where to find the heart sounds while taking a blood pressure reading. When a patient called her "Doctor," she laughed out loud.

At Douglas Moore, the residents didn't know her history with RAMP. They didn't know that she almost needed to remediate a committee or that she harbored fantasies of being a part-time housewife. They saw an eager young woman who wanted to do what they were doing, help people who were invisible to other people. In this clinic, patients had chronic health problems complicated by old age. The residents went out of their way to help her, and Gentry finally got the one-on-one patient contact she craved.

A few times at Douglas Moore, her preceptor listened as she presented patients, but Gentry didn't feel comfortable around her. Because Gentry got so much help from the residents, she didn't mind that her preceptor seemed uninterested in her progress. Besides, her preceptor's office door was often closed. Gentry didn't go out of her way to get to know the woman behind it.

Although the RAMP experience made Gentry work harder, she still strove for competency, not excellence. "I don't want to be a superstar or the chair of a department," she told me. "What good are these things if I [have to] go have dinner alone and I have no one to shop with?" Statements like these made her stand out from her peers, often overachievers who seemed to really care about impressing people. I worried Gentry's comments made her seem shallow, and I hoped she wasn't just giving me sound bites that would please a reality TV show producer. One weekend evening, I got her on the phone around 10 P.M., and I finally told her I didn't understand her. "Why do you act like you don't care when I know you care deeply about becoming a good doctor?"

She didn't disagree with that statement. She just listened to the case I was making. Like Franco, she often noted health-care disparities based on ethnic background, socioeconomic status, and gender—especially gender. She told me that having seen so many young women's lives derailed by teenage pregnancy in her small, overwhelmingly Catholic and Hispanic hometown, she'd decided to devote as much time as she could supporting abortion rights. She even trained to be a patient escort at a local abortion clinic in addition to leading Medical Students for Choice on the Case campus. Gentry worried about her performance constantly, often getting so nervous before presentations and exams that she couldn't sleep the night before.

We talked for a long time that night. By the end of our conversation, I had had no startling insights, just that sometimes she didn't get herself either.

During Gentry's preceptorship, she did her first breast exam. It was on an eighty-four-year-old woman, not the easiest sort of patient. Her breasts were long and slack, and Gentry tried her best to put her at ease as she examined every inch of them. Naturally curious, she got patients to give her exactly the kind of information she needed most of the time. After a while, Gentry became more confident taking histories. She got a new piercing through the middle of her ear. She even started dating someone—a second-year student who'd crashed Franco's potluck back in the winter just to see her. Things seemed to be getting better. She was doing things, seeing real patients.

"After spending countless hours chained to [my] desk, endeavoring to learn how to spell words like pancreaticoduodenal and uvulopalatopharyngoplasty (words I don't actually know how to spell but do know how to copy from a medical dictionary), it is difficult for me to explain why I chose to become a doctor," she wrote in a reflection paper about her preceptorship on November 28, 2006. "Yet after time spent at places like Douglas Moore, I am reminded why I continue to study, and just how much I have to learn."

Gentry finished her preceptorship at the Douglas Moore clinic in the spring of 2007. She thanked the residents and left the clinic thinking it was the best experience of med school so far. As she was preparing for the third year, what med students often recall as the hardest, her society dean, Robert Haynie, called her into his office. "There are all these concerns about you," he told her.

Her review—submitted by the preceptor she rarely saw—was scathing. She was "selfish." That was the word her preceptor had used to describe how she presented patient cases at the Douglas Moore clinic. Also, her skirts were too short, and she was more interested in socializing than patient care. Gentry was floored. She told Haynie she hadn't known her preceptor felt that way about her; she'd never told Gentry any of this. Perhaps she did wear a shorter-than-acceptable skirt. Why hadn't anyone told her? Gentry saw whatever patients the resident she was shadowing saw. Should she have asked to see more? Again, why hadn't anyone told her? And the comment about the patient presentations? Yeah, that was probably right. But again, why didn't she say something?

Gentry listened to Haynie. He gave her advice: be diplomatic. Think about how what you say will reflect on you, and don't say anything bad about anyone you work with. If some part of the program doesn't live up to your expectations, tell the people who can change it. Don't complain about it to everyone else. In short, be professional. She agreed to set up a meeting with the preceptor, to show that she was receptive to her comments, to show that she cared about becoming a good physician. Maybe there was a chance the preceptor would temper her comments. It was one thing to blow off reflection papers; it was much worse to get trashed in a formal review. And this was a clinical experience where she saw real patients, one where *she* thought she learned some things.

As Gentry walked away from Haynie's office, the anger set in. She should not have been blindsided by the preceptor's comments. That, Gentry felt, was not fair. The preceptor was unprofessional too.

The Boards

Less than an hour before she was to take the hardest exam of her life, I found Gentry kneeling in her kitchen cupboard, searching for a plastic container for oatmeal. The instant variety had become a staple of her diet, easily prepared and consumed under the diagram of kidney function in her kitchen or beneath the whiteboard at school where she drew viruses.

Gentry was hungry, and she needed to eat something. While attempting to make eggs at 3 A.M., she'd nearly set the pharmacology flash card for clindamycin on fire when she turned on the wrong burner. She really did want to see her study materials go up in flames, but she had too much to prove before purging. This test—step 1 of the United States Medical Licensing Examination (USMLE), otherwise known as the boards—is an eight-hour marathon of specimen identification, graph interpretation, and clinical problem-solving covering anatomy, pathology, microbiology, and much more.

I remembered the defiant and easily distracted med student Gentry used to be, the one who pulled me into a trinket shop in Chinatown to look for Halloween costumes when we were supposed to be having an interview, the one who bragged about investigating modeling opportunities when she should have been studying. She was no longer that student. It was not the blistering review from the preceptor she didn't respect that changed her, nor the stern lecture from the society dean she did respect. It was this test. While studying for boards, she did not clean, she did not shop, and she did not go out with friends. This test made her realize that she could not have a life while pursuing the knowledge she needed to practice medicine. It must become an all-encompassing endeavor. Before she could burn her notes, she needed a good step 1 score to prove how serious she was about medicine. More importantly, she needed it to secure a residency in dermatology, one of the most sought-after specialties.

The theme song from *Rocky* boomed out of Gentry's cell phone. It was a med school friend. "Take some Tylenol with caffeine," she said. "You can't cancel now."

She and Gentry were taking the boards on March 24, 2007, one week late. They'd delayed it as long as they could, and their third-year rotations were about to start. In the third year, the students would apply what they'd learned to clinical settings. But first, they had to take this test. They had to prove they'd mastered enough science behind the practice of medicine.

Gentry's professors didn't teach to the boards, so during a six-week break from classes, she crammed complicated nerve pathways, random side effects, and odds ratios in between bouts of distraction, the inevitable result of perusing so many illustrated medical texts (a nose consumed by fungi in blastomycosis, a body infested with pinworms).

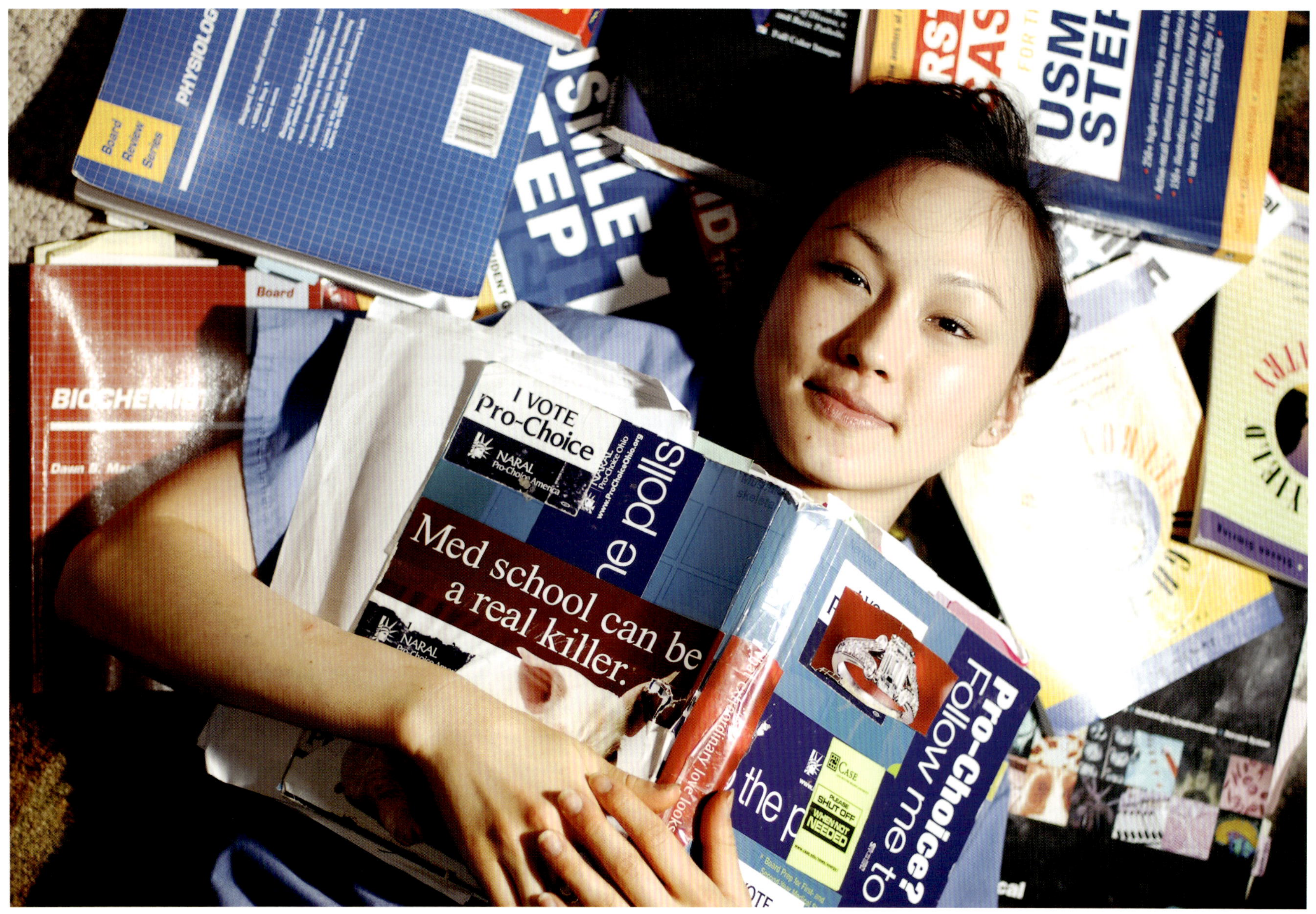

Gentry spent her second year studying for the boards. In summer 2007, she posed with some of the books she used to prepare for the test that would make—or break—her chances at getting a residency in radiology, one of the most sought-after specialties.

She hadn't studied enough path or pharm, of that she was sure. She hadn't wasted much time on anatomy. She was hoping for questions on genetic diseases, which she'd studied extensively because they're interesting and easy (treatment: nothing, prognosis: death).

At 7:30 A.M., the oatmeal was packed, the vitamin B pills were swallowed, and Gentry's tote bag and worn blue backpack with the broken zipper were straining under the weight of study guides, Coke, and Red Bull.

"I'll be amazed if I don't puke," she said, climbing into my car.

Gentry and her friend didn't say much during the drive to the testing site, which was about forty minutes away in the suburb of Stow, near Akron. They looked tired—beat, really—still working toward acceptance of the fact that I would not be turning the car around. (In fact, because of our slow start, I was driving as fast as I could without attracting the traffic cops.) This test was going to happen. There was nothing they could do to stop it now.

The testing site was a tan storefront next to a Wal-Mart and a Lowe's and across the street from a Dollar Tree. Gentry walked into the waiting room, with its mauve chairs and mauve doors and mauve carpeting, and gave a man at the window her ID, then she popped some Tylenol and plopped down on the floor underneath a picture that read, "The tougher the challenge, the greater the triumph."

Despite an unfortunate affinity for the dark pink shade commonly paired with gray in the 1980s, whoever designed the room had intended for it to be a calming place. But the waiting room was having the opposite effect on Gentry. She was panicking, thinking of all the things she wished she had done that might have made this moment more bearable. If only she had more money, she could have taken the Kaplan course. If only she had been more organized, she could have taken the test earlier. If only. If only. If only. She felt resigned. She felt like she would die. She felt resigned again. What she knew, she knew. That was all.

She took a few sips of Red Bull, checking the vitamin B content. She flipped through a study guide. On the cover, she had taped the sentence "Med School Can Kill You" next to a picture of an engagement ring and a pro-choice sticker.

"Millicent," the man at the window said. "Let's get you up."

She stalled a moment more, flipping through the guide. Reluctantly, she rose, throwing her backpack over one shoulder and her tote filled with caffeinated beverages over the other. She opened the door with great difficulty and passed through it.

•◆◆•

The pass rate for first-time step 1 test takers at U.S. and Canadian medical schools was 94 percent in 2005, and 95 percent in 2006, according to the National Board of Medical Examiners. Dr. Daniel B. Ornt, vice dean for education and academic affairs at Case, told me that Case's pass rate is near 100 percent, so most students aren't worried about failing. They're worried about doing better than the other test takers. The higher their score, the greater the likelihood they will land a residency in the most competitive, best-paying specialties, such as neurosurgery, orthopedics, plastic surgery, ENT (ear, nose, and throat), ophthalmology, and dermatology. Even for less competitive fields, if students are pursuing well-regarded and highly appealing residency programs, the scores count. Case administrators say students aspiring to residencies in competitive fields or at highly sought-after programs must score at or even one standard deviation above the national mean of 220 to get an interview. The applications of students who receive lower scores may not be reviewed at all. If anything, the scores have become more important, even though, as the authors of a recent Carnegie Foundation report remind us, a poor correlation exists between step 1 scores and supervisor ratings during residency.

Some have bemoaned the high-stakes reputation of the boards. Students know residency programs use step 1 scores to help determine their competitiveness, so they focus on the test at the expense of other learning—not to mention their health, relationships, and sanity-preserving personal interests. In the few weeks before the boards, it was hard for me to get the students on the phone. When I did, they seemed completely ensconced in their studying. In March 2007, the Iraq War was heating up. Tornadoes ravaged the southern states. *Playboy* founder Hugh Hefner turned eighty-one. But nothing in the news—or their personal lives—distracted them for long.

One Sunday morning a few weeks before the boards, Franco woke up to a spinning room and a reeling stomach. She leaned over the side of the bed and threw up. When she turned her head, she threw up again. She remembered the neurology she'd studied. Something was wrong with her inner ear. Without moving her head, she reached for her cell phone and called her mentor, Bob, who assured her it wasn't an "acoustic neuroma" (tumor). He thought it was a virus. For a second opinion, she called society dean Haynie. He told her he also thought it was a virus. She then called student health services. A nurse there told her it was probably a virus.

Franco lay face down in her bed for hours. Finally, she got up to go to the health clinic. On her way down the stairs, she threw up twice, both times on her boyfriend. The worry welled up in her. How long would this last? How could she study? What if she got sick during the boards?

For the next several weeks, she endured more throwing up and a shot of a potent anti-vomiting medication followed by the same drug in pill form. She went through the symptoms as if she were confronting a question on the boards: dizziness, nausea, nystagmus (a condition that causes the eyes to twitch in their sockets). But unlike with the board questions, she couldn't check a text or ask a doctor friend for the answer. No one knew how to fix her.

Franco was very sick, but she couldn't stop worrying about the boards. The immense stress that step 1 inflicts on students is not the only or even the biggest focus of criticism of the exam. Its timing (at the end of the second year) impedes radical curriculum reorganization—the kind of reorganization some believe necessary for medical education to keep pace with societal needs and expectations. Step 1 covers basic sciences that schools are expected to teach students in their first two years, and schools can veer from that only at their students' peril. If students don't know the material, they won't score competitively. While the authors of the Carnegie report note that attention to the "core competencies necessary for medical practice has sparked efforts to rethink the examinations required for licensure," they don't know if any changes will occur.

Although I found plenty of academic griping about step 1—it came nowhere close to the level of student griping I witnessed—no one has advocated eliminating licensure tests altogether. America had a standardless medical profession long ago, and it was a dark age to which medical educators hope never to return. In the American colonies, there were no legal standards of proficiency or control of medical practice. In the 1840s in northern Ohio, a preceptor just needed to file a certificate of proficiency with the local town clerk or probate judge, and his former student would then be able to start seeing patients on his own. By about 1920, just a decade after Flexner's report was published, the medical profession had developed accreditation, certification, and licensing procedures to monitor medical schools and protect patients. The National Board of Medical Examiners established the NBME Part Examination, designed to test medical students' competency. In the early 1990s, the USMLE replaced it, as well as the Federation of State Medical Boards Licensing Examination. The USMLE spans the four years of medical school and the first year of residency, called the internship. Again, students take step 1 at the end of their second year in medical school. They take step 2, which tests their ability to apply their clinical knowledge and skills to patient-care settings, in their fourth year. This test involves a "performance" portion, where the students are assessed as they take histories and examine and talk with standardized patients (actors pretending to be patients). Step 3 is taken during or after the internship year, depending on the state. It tests physicians' knowledge and its application to clinical practice. It is the final assessment before doctors assume "independent responsibility" in delivering medical care. According to USMLE, candidates should pass all three steps within seven years.

Of the three parts of the USMLE, step 1—because it is the first and the most imperative to residency—seems to be the most nerve wracking. Researchers have shown there's little evidence that taking commercial preparatory courses improves step 1 scores, but students spend hundreds or thousands on them anyway. They pore over guidebooks such as *First Aid* and pay Kaplan hundreds of dollars for access to its QBank, an online database of USMLE-type questions and explanations of answers.

In between bites of a turkey wrap, Norton studied a question from the Kaplan QBank, which he'd bought along with Kaplan Web-Prep for $1,100, money he'd saved by eventually opting out of the Case student medical plan and getting on Medicaid along with his wife and daughter:

> A 62-year-old man with severe shortness of breath undergoes a lung biopsy that reveals diffuse disposition of calcium into the pulmonary interstitium. Which of the following diseases is most likely to produce this type of severe metastatic calcification?
>
> A) Amyloidosis
> B) Goodpasture's Syndrome
> C) Hypoparathyroidism
> D) Medullary carcinoma
> E) Multiple myeloma

Norton chose E, the correct answer. He got many of the QBank questions right that day in March 2007, which he spent mostly by himself in a study room at school. But he was still worried about the test he'd be taking in a few days.

I asked him why.

"It's the uncertainty of how it's going to turn out," he said, picking the peppers out of his sandwich.

Science's goal is to eliminate as much uncertainty as possible, and Norton is a man of science. Uncertainty bothers him—he can't even read a book without skipping to the end to make sure the hero lives. Perhaps that was one reason he filled his life with as many fixed variables as possible: Kate, the always patient and supportive wife who held the same values; the Mormon religion he was born into

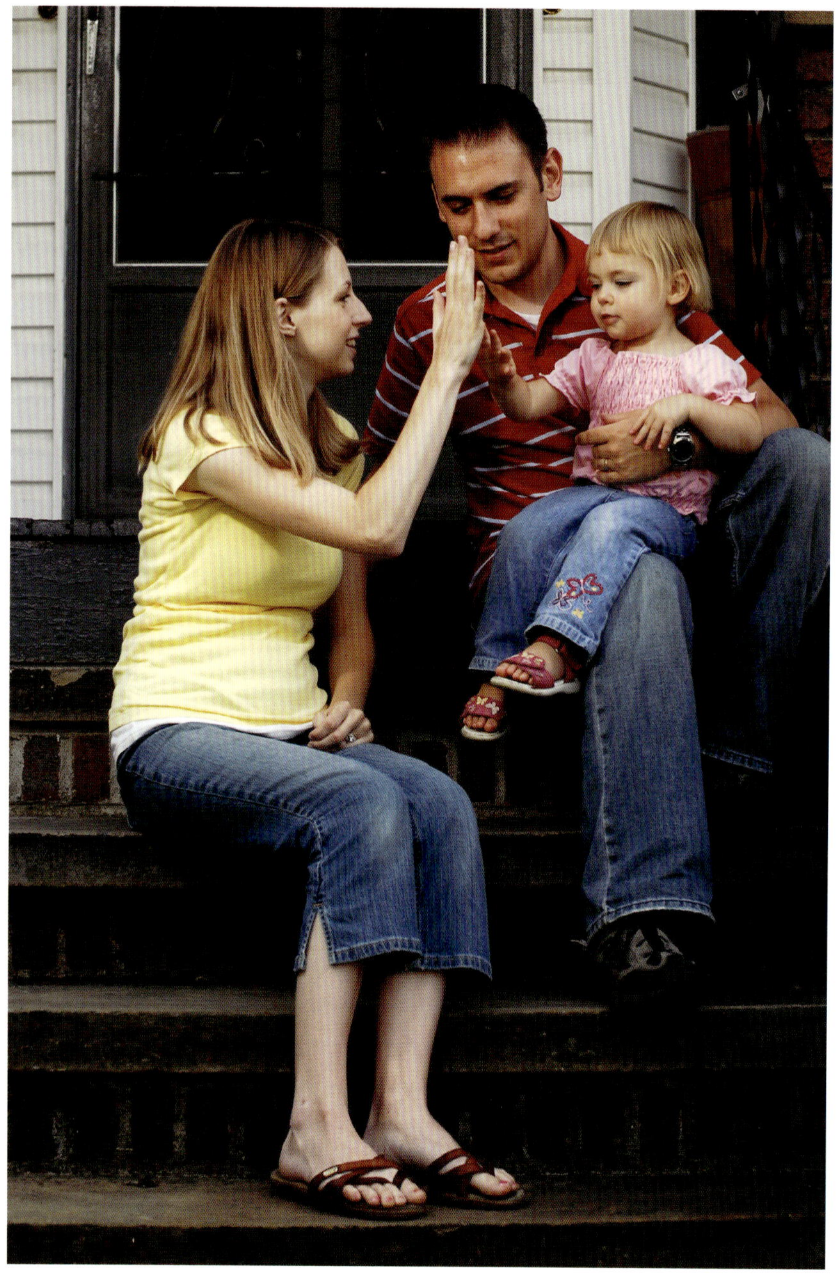

and believed deeply in; and eighteen-month-old Megan and (quite possibly) a new baby on the way, the first two children of the big family he had always wanted.

There was comfort for Norton in knowing what he's good at, who loves him, and why he's here on earth. It baffled him that lesser issues, such as this test, could fill him with so much anxiety. He saw a biochemistry question he didn't know the answer to and he thought, *I don't know anything!* Then he looked up the answer. He'd probably remember it forever, he said. He knew there'd be other questions, ones he'd never seen, on the test too. No matter how much studying he did, the test would be an ordeal of uncertainty.

He took comfort in a quote from his favorite TV show, *Scrubs:* "OK, you're scared. That's good. That's what makes you not a crappy doctor." Or a crappy med student.

Norton treated studying for the boards like a job. He got up at 7 A.M., got to school by 8, and studied there until 6:30 P.M., which gave him an hour to play with Megan before she went to bed. Sometimes Kate brought Megan to see him at school and she cried when it was time to leave. He worried that he neglected his family, but overall he thought their support—which he defined as everything from dinner to goodnight kisses—outweighed the negatives. "I look at my classmates and wonder how they do it without a family," he said.

Norton didn't worry about earning a 185, the passing score on the boards. (The average is between 200 and 220.) He wanted to score in the 230s or, even better, the 240s, which would make him competitive for everything, including cardiology and pulmonology, the specialties he was considering.

Norton, Kate, and Megan share some unscheduled time on the front porch of their rented duplex in June 2007.

He studied by reading review books, watching Kaplan online audio lectures, and taking practice tests, as many as four a day. He talked about the test all the time. When he mentioned it, Kate rolled her eyes. "You're worried about by how big a margin you're going to pass, not whether you're going to pass," she reminded him.

The day before the test, he focused on studying antibiotics and anticancer drugs in between episodes of *Scrubs.* At night, he, Kate, and Megan went to Dairy Queen and splurged on Blizzards. Being $110,000 in debt for med school already, they didn't go out much. But after four weeks of dealing with this test, he figured they all deserved a treat.

Really, not being able to afford treats was the least of it. The three of them depended on the state for food stamps and medical care. When Norton needed a root canal, his parents had to help him pay for it. Kate never complained about having to dress Megan in secondhand clothes, but Norton wanted them to have more.

When he saw an Army recruiter posting flyers in the medical school, Norton stopped and asked him for more information. He learned that if he joined the Army as an officer, the government would pay for his education. It would give him training at an Army hospital after medical school or, if no military residency was available in the specialty he chose, allow him to compete for a civilian one. Army residents make $60,000 a year, much more than what most residents earn at civilian hospitals. He would owe the Army one year for every year of residency. For instance, if he did a two-year family practice residency, he'd owe them two years. If he chose to stay in longer, the Army would take over the loans he'd incurred during his first two years of medical school.

Norton wouldn't be the first in his family to join the military. His mother's father won a Bronze Star in the Battle of the Bulge and his father's father got a Purple Heart after being burned by a phosphorus grenade in World War II while helping a buddy out of danger. Joining the Army would be a great thing on every front, Norton reasoned, except one.

The war.

He talked more to the recruiter, who assured him that after spending so much money to train him, the Army would do everything possible to keep him out of danger, even if he were sent to Iraq. But Norton said he didn't have a problem being deployed; he just didn't want a deployment to interrupt his residency. Norton also talked to other medical students in the armed forces, as well as Army doctors. He talked to Kate about it, for months, and she never rolled her eyes. His father said what he always said. *Weigh your options. Don't do it for financial reasons. Make sure it's what you really want to do.*

Although he himself never enlisted, Norton's father raised his two sons and two daughters always to respect the military. He was raised on the west side of Salt Lake City. In his youth, he was a bit of a troublemaker. He and his brothers used to make slingshots out of rubber bands and hit cars with crab apples until they accidently hit a police car. They would put coal on the railroad tracks until the conductor showed up at their house. Norton loved hearing these stories because they showed another version of his dad, a less perfect version, one that gave him hope that he could grow into someone as good as his father someday.

His father graduated from the University of Utah with degrees in computer science and Spanish literature. He moved his young family to Portland, Oregon, in 1988. In the mid-1990s, he went into marketing after getting his MBA. He worked hard, but he was almost always home for dinner. He made sure he spent time with his family every night.

Norton often called him for advice, and lately, the boards were providing a good distraction from an even bigger problem weighing on Norton's mind. For months, Bryan Norton had felt weakness in his hands. A few weeks before Christmas 2006, doctors ruled out carpal tunnel syndrome. Soon after that, I gave Norton a ride home from school. He was telling me about how he'd sawed open the skull of his group's cadaver with a special drill with a half-moon blade. He'd tried not to inhale the fine dust particles of bone as he drilled, being careful not to slice into the brain. When he finally succeeded in pulling the skull back, he stared at the brain, amazed at how electrical impulses can turn into pain or sight or taste in that mushy thing.

"They're all just neurons firing," he said. "But they're all different. How do they turn into memory? It's incredible. It's one of the reasons I'm considering neuro."

He suddenly stopped talking for a moment and lowered his voice.

"Please don't print this," he said.

"Of course I won't," I said.

His father's doctors knew he didn't have carpal tunnel because other nerves outside the hand and arm were involved. Norton had been researching his father's symptoms, and he came up with a worst-case diagnosis: amyotrophic lateral sclerosis.

I didn't know much about ALS, just that it is about as bad a diagnosis as someone can get. (It's also known as Lou Gehrig's disease, after the New York Yankees baseball legend who died of ALS in 1941.) If you have this disease, you eventually lose the ability to control your muscles, but it doesn't affect the brain. The electrical impulses in the brain, that amazing organ, just keep firing as usual. You continue to see and hear and feel and make memories as you progressively lose the ability to move your body. Eventually you lose the ability to speak, to cough, and, eventually, to breathe. Patients die of it, Norton said, usually within five years of diagnosis.

For once, Norton didn't rush to fill the silence between us. He didn't want to talk about it anymore.

The Wards

Unshaven and looking as eager as he could on three hours' sleep, Norton paced a long, narrow hallway of the Cleveland Clinic where patients awaited surgical consultations. A surgeon he was not, not yet—maybe not ever, if his wife got her way. But in September 2007, five weeks into his third-year surgical rotation, Norton wondered if he could be happy doing anything else.

Yesterday he'd helped suction blood out of a woman whose aorta—the largest vessel carrying blood from the heart—was bleeding into her abdomen. Also torn were the tissue-like walls of her inferior vena cava—a major vein carrying blood to the heart. Blood pooled in the patient's abdomen as fast as Norton could suction it. The sutures threatened to tear through the walls. But the surgeon kept working, snipping, slicing and sewing, fixing her.

During this rotation another surgeon told Norton, "We're the same as other doctors, except two days a week, we get to go to the playground." Norton already understood completely.

As a third-year medical student, he knew how to tie knots like the Eagle Scout he'd once been, place nasal gastric tubes and Foley catheters, even drive the little camera in laparoscopic surgery. He found every surgery endlessly fascinating, from a simple hernia repair to the complicated (and hard-to-pronounce) pancreaticoduodenectomy. The OR was "fun," the surgeons "amazing." The details stuck in his head, and he recounted them later, slice by slice, if I asked. Interspersed in all his enthusiasm, however, was doubt about his potential. He still hadn't managed to impress Dr. R. Matthew Walsh, a general surgeon who specializes in pancreatic surgery and the one in charge on the day I shadowed him in surgery clinic.

During back-to-back gallbladder surgeries, Walsh pummeled Norton with questions about cholangitis, an inflammation of the bile ducts that both patients suffered from. He followed up Norton's answers with "Are you sure?" Again and again. "Are you sure?" When Norton was wrong, a new line of questions followed. When he was right, a new line of questions followed.

Norton was among those medical students who aced most of their exams (even step 1 of the boards) and easily picked up the physical part of being a physician. They get used to smiles of appreciation from their instructors, who describe them as "motivated" on evaluations, and their performance as "thorough." They thrive under the kinder, gentler instruction of the modern medical school.

But Walsh is not an instructor for the self-esteem junkies of Norton's generation. If surgery is the playground, some might see him as the bully. But is it bullying or conditioning? That depends on if you can take it.

When Walsh emerged from a patient room, a tall, elegant figure with a surgeon's slight stoop, Norton snapped to attention. Walsh was indifferent to him, writing something.

"Mike, do you have something to do?" Walsh asked without looking up.

"I'm preparing to see Mrs. B——?"

Mrs. B——'s online chart said her condition was "not disclosed via Dr. Cosgrove."

"I should see her," Walsh said at first. Toby Cosgrove is CEO and president of the Cleveland Clinic. In Norton's mind, the patient had VIP status, and he was not surprised that Walsh didn't want to bother her with a med student.

Then Walsh changed his mind and told Norton to see her first.

"I saw Dr. Cosgrove's name and thought you might want to see her yourself . . ."

Walsh waved him off as he walked down the hall.

Unlike the first two years of medical school, the third requires some weight-pulling in real clinical settings. Even though the students' work is double-checked by doctors, they still have a place on the team. Expectations must be met beyond learning more about medicine. Histories must be taken, physical exams given, and presentations and assessments made. Above all else, medical students don't want to look like idiots. Next, they want to be useful. They are told they are part of the team, and they want to act like it.

Several doctors and medical educators I interviewed used the term "rite of passage" to describe a student's time on the wards, as if third year is a transition for the future doctor, like puberty or marriage, only with its own distinct rites. In his landmark work, *Les Rites de Passage,* the French anthropologist Arnold van Gennep explained that "the life of an individual in any society is a series of passages from one age to another and from one occupation to another." Wherever there are distinctions among groups—such as medical students, residents, and attending physicians, for instance—there are special acts that accompany ascension to the higher group. Van Gennep broke these acts into three phases. The first is separation, when a person begins withdrawing from his or her original group. The second is transition, a difficult period of limbo between two groups. Rites associated with this phase are called "liminal rites." Finally, there is incorporation, when a person enters the new group.

Third year is definitely the liminal year. There are no normal days, no real confidence, just the fleeting sort one gets from a preceptor's satisfied look. The transition that students make during their third year would be easier if the students spent more time in each service, getting familiar with the culture and the personalities. But at Case Med, the third year is characterized by short stints in the major services: internal medicine, surgery, family medicine, pediatrics, obstetrics and gynecology, neurology, and psychiatry. The students complete two sixteen-week blocks during which they do clinical work, and one sixteen-week block during which they do research, which is a feature of the school's new curriculum. Norton's class had the most clinical experience of any third-year class to date. But it didn't seem to make things easier for him.

He entered the room of the VIP patient. About a half hour later he came out and started pacing again, studying a note card he'd pulled out of the bulging pockets of his white coat. He spotted Walsh.

"I'm ready whenever you are," Norton called.

"You're totally ready."

Walsh disappeared into another patient room, leaving Norton to obsess over his presentation for a few more minutes.

"It doesn't matter how thorough I am," he said quietly. "Walsh will be more so."

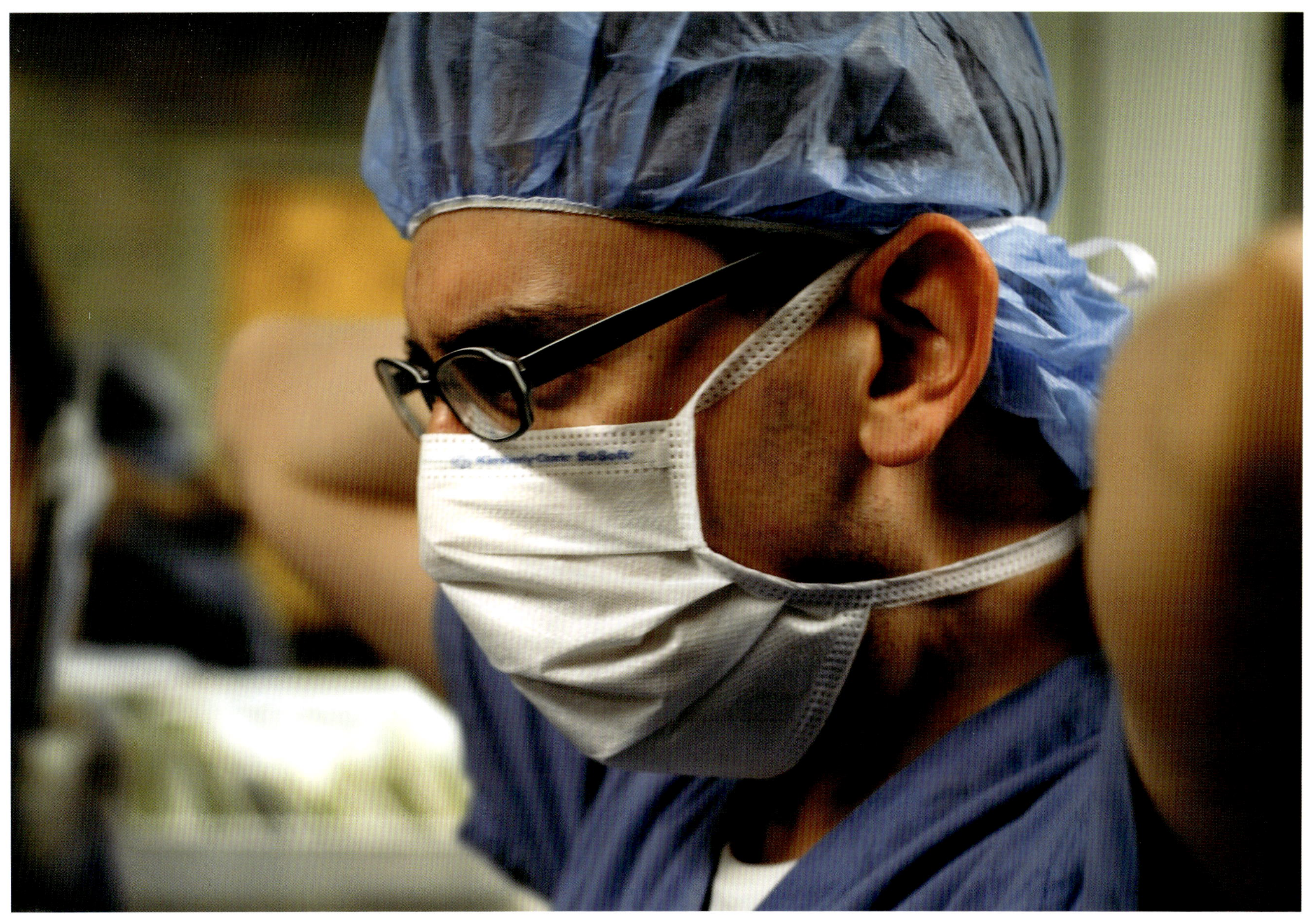

Norton loved his third-year surgery rotation—it challenged him more than any other experience in medical school. But he suspected the demands of that specialty would be in direct conflict with his parenting. How could he be both a surgeon and the dad he always wanted to be?

The surgeon flipped through a chart as Norton began. "She plans her life around eating and going to the bathroom." Walsh asked about her allergies, her meds, her history of gallbladder disease, whether her colon was enlarged. He asked Norton to tell him everything causing her pain, if she had cirrhosis.

"If I take her gallbladder and she has cirrhosis, what's the chance she could die?" Walsh asked.

"I don't know," Norton confessed.

"Eighty percent."

After more questions, Norton followed Walsh into the patient's room, his forehead shiny with sweat. When he came back out twenty minutes later, Norton looked shaken.

Walsh left him standing there thinking about why he didn't tell him about the C-section scar or the severe and persistent pain in the right upper quadrant of the patient's abdomen.

Disappointment spread across Norton's face like a rash.

• ◆ ◆ •

On an elevator at the Miller Family Heart & Vascular Institute of the Cleveland Clinic in May 2007, Gentry practiced her presentation. She had an intern's pager number written on her arm and the book *Pocket Brain: EKG and Heart Murmurs* tucked into the pocket of her white coat.

None of the students wanted me to publish their scores on step 1. But Gentry said she did "OK." That anxiety seemed ancient to her now. It was her second day with Dr. Richard Krasuski, an attending physician at the nation's #1 heart program, according to *U.S. News and World Report,* and she needed to not blow it. She couldn't have had a more helpful patient, a smart, talkative thirty-one-year-old single woman who said she ran a few miles three days a week. She went to her local hospital after getting chest pain that lasted all day, got better, then seemed to turn into bad upper gastrointestinal pain. Routine tests yielded nothing helpful. When they wanted to do a heart catheterization, an invasive procedure, she came here.

Yesterday, Gentry had spent a long time with the patient and her parents. Today, the patient complained about being awakened six times during the night and giving the nurses what seemed like gallons of her blood. Gentry smiled sympathetically and listened to her heart. Sounded good to her, but she was still learning to listen to heart sounds. One cardiologist told her you have to hear something hundreds of times to know what it is.

On the eleventh floor, Krasuski's team gathered around a too-small table. Like Gentry, some had been there all night, handling patients who ranged from Gentry's seemingly healthy young woman to a lifelong smoker. In their heads were stats and studies, social and physical histories, and questions for Krasuski, a Harvard Medical School graduate with a gentle, well-mannered way that belied a fierce intellect.

Members of the team took turns presenting. Krasuski, an expert in adult congenital heart disease, listened, questioned, and offered insight, usually in that order. He asked the most questions of Gentry, who maintained her calm demeanor, which some mistake for aloofness, even when she admitted she had no idea what answer he was looking for.

"Oh, man," she said in response to a drug-related question. "I'm blanking because I'm under stress."

"You can ask for a consult from a pharmacist," Krasuski offered.

It went on like this for more than two hours.

Medical students call a physician's willful infliction of humiliation on their kind "pimping." But Dr. Dan Wolpaw, a Case professor of medicine in charge of the clinical curriculum, explained that questioning is necessary in order to "diagnose the learner"—to find out what a student knows and how to help her learn what she doesn't. True pimping still happens, but not nearly as much as it used to.

At the end of the meeting, they still didn't have a diagnosis for Gentry's patient. Every test she took was fine except one. It might have been a false positive. But Krasuski said there was a slim chance she could have acute coronary syndrome. He decided she needed one more test in order to rule it out.

For the rest of rounds, Gentry followed Krasuski in and out of patient rooms, observing his bedside manner, which was both pleasant and intense. "Can I have a quick listen?" was how he asked patients to let him listen to their chests. "I know you've already gone through a lot" was how he asked them for just one more test. Even though his phone rang every few minutes—he was in charge of approving transfers to the hospital that day—often requiring him to duck out of the room, he didn't forget Gentry. When he took a quick listen, he made sure she did too.

"Lead the way," he told her at one point. "You're the doctor."

•◆◆◆•

Franco did not throw up during the boards, on which she scored below average, she said. She also got a diagnosis—ear infections in both ears—but it didn't completely explain the vertigo, which persisted on and off for months. During her first third-year rotation—in surgery—she had to force herself to get out of bed to be at the hospital by 5:45 A.M.

"Surgeons are some of the briskest people I've ever met," she told me. It's a high-stress culture, one she already knew she didn't want to be part of. Yet for four weeks she was required to immerse herself in it. In the OR, a strange, sterile world, she felt as vulnerable as the patient lying on the table, skin retracted, organs exposed—only she was awake. Sometimes she couldn't speak. During rounds, she hung back and let other students answer the attending physician's questions. She assisted in surgeries that lasted from one to six hours, which crept by as she stood, holding retractors. She found surgeons liked to drill med students holding retractors.

Her first surgery was a hernia repair, and she had trouble answering a question about hernia reoccurrence rates. "That's the worst answer I've ever gotten," the surgeon told her, and she had to fight back tears. Even when she thought she knew the answer to a question someone asked her in surgery, it didn't always make its way out of her mouth. The surgical mask felt like a gag. She tried to blame intermittent vertigo and exhaustion—sometimes her beeper went off so often she got less than an hour of sleep over a twenty-four-hour period. But there was something else to her speechlessness, too—and this was what really scared her. She still felt inadequate, like she didn't know enough to be there, like she'd never know enough.

Franco saw many surgeries for hernias and appendicitis during the rotation, so she learned a lot about those conditions. When she got home from the hospital after 6 P.M., she read studies and reviewed her notes from the first two years. She was surprised by how much bowel she saw in the OR. One patient's diseased colon actually spilled out all over her and others on the surgery team. *Shit,* she thought, *I'm covered in shit.*

One day in April 2007, an attending physician pricked Franco's double-gloved hand with a scalpel. She saw blood—or was it just a nightmare mirage of the OR? She rushed out of the OR to the nurse's station. When she pulled her gloves off, more blood flowed from the pinprick, and the dam burst on her emotions. Unlike the first time she cried in the OR, this time she didn't care who heard her. She bawled as they took her blood for the rapid HIV test.

This was shit.

· ◆ ◆ ◆ ·

Gentry spent four dollars on a paperback, *A Brief History of Art,* at Borders, and she read from it nearly every day. Ever since she'd moved to Cleveland, she'd wanted to visit the Cleveland Museum of Art, one of the city's renowned cultural institutions. But it had been undergoing a massive expansion, and much of the museum was closed for renovation. In early November 2007, the fall of her third year at Case, the Modern Masters exhibit was finally open. It featured European paintings and sculptures from the late nineteenth and early twentieth centuries, and Gentry looked forward to sampling the museum's impressive collection of Cézannes and Van Goghs.

We visited the museum together on a Saturday. Gentry was a good art museum companion, present and perceptive but not too chatty. She liked Degas' dancer drawings. ("So much skill," she said). She knew the difference between a Manet and a Monet. We stopped in front of Monet's water lilies. It is a large work, and you have to stand fairly far back in order to take it all in. I know why people like impressionism; it invites them to see what they want to see. I like to see what is, but the painting appealed to Gentry, so I stood next to her looking at all those blurry flowers and lily pads and other pond life. Perhaps because they resemble the edgeless images of tumors and fractures, Gentry started talking about radiology.

Although she hadn't dismissed dermatology as a specialty yet, she said radiology appealed to her visual nature. Radiologists spend a lot of time looking at images, solving problems for people they may never have to meet. (If you never have to meet them, they can't judge the way you speak or act.) There's no one-upmanship with other doctors. They're collaborators, consultants. They get to diagnose the fracture or the tumor, but you don't have to "manage the patient."

The word "manage" stuck in my head. Why did she use that word instead of "treat" or "follow"? At times, the students parroted terms they'd heard others use, and I wasn't sure if the meanings they carried in the nonmedical world were the ones they intended. "Managing" patients doesn't sound noble, and I don't think I'd ever heard it on a doctor drama. The character traits I most respected in Gentry—her independence, her honesty, her dedication—rarely seemed to come through in my writing as much as laziness, self-centeredness, and apathy, traits she seemed to hold because of her words more than her actions. To me, she was real. But I worried that to my readers she seemed undeserving of the white coat. Doctors are supposed to be committed to saving the world, not making it to yoga class on time. Because of her preoccupations and her frankness, even her activism, Gentry was the most millennial of the three doctors-to-be I followed.

It's common for medical students to change their career plans during or after the third year, when they encounter a variety of specialists in many different settings. Reality often ends the romance with surgery or emergency medicine, the darlings of television producers, while inspiring new fascinations with specialties students never considered before. Although Gentry's cardiology rotation at the Cleveland Clinic went well, Krasuski told me later that she wasn't one of the top students he'd seen—she could have done more research on her own and been more inquisitive. But he said she did "reasonably well." He added, "You look for how they interact with patients, and she did a very nice job with this young lady [her patient]."

On the first day of her surgery rotation, Gentry found out her cat died. Then one surgeon grilled her so hard she started crying in front of him. ("If you told me I had to be a surgeon, I'd be a waitress," she told me later.) The next day, she was supposed to follow a different surgeon, but he told her he was too busy. No problem, she told him, secretly relieved to get out of surgery clinic. She'd just get some studying done instead. While sitting at a computer in the Cleveland Clinic Breast Center, she saw a woman in heels and a flowing rose-print red dress. Gentry started talking with her. The woman was a medical breast specialist who took time off to raise her children. She had just gotten back into medicine. Did Gentry want to sit in on a consult?

Gentry couldn't believe her luck. For three years, she'd been looking for someone like her—a doctor who didn't just talk about the importance of taking time for yourself and your family. Here was someone who actually did it. And she was employed. And she was offering to show Gentry a few things. Gentry could have skipped over to the patient room with her.

The patient was a middle-aged woman with a dime-sized lump in her breast. Gentry listened carefully to the interview and watched the specialist examine her. But even after all that, she couldn't determine if it was cancer without an ultrasound. So Gentry followed the patient to the imaging room. That's where Gentry met a radiologist, Dr. Christine Quinn. She ran an ultrasound probe over the patient's breast. Amorphous black-and-white blobs appeared on the screen as Gentry watched, rapt.

"I know what this is," Quinn told the patient. A benign mass, possibly something left from the patient's breast implants. Definitely not cancer. The patient's expression of concern morphed into relief. In that dark room, Gentry found her future specialty. Quinn was a problem solver, as well as a compassionate doctor and a really nice person. She was who Gentry wanted to be one day.

She just didn't know if the competitive radiology specialty would want her.

•◆◆•

In June 2007, Franco got to work at the Thomas F. McCafferty Health Center, which had actually been her first choice (which she didn't get) for a second-year preceptorship because of the clinic's largely Hispanic patient base. Her first patient of the day was Delia, a smiley ten-year-old girl with hair down to her waist and two stickers, rewards for the six shots she'd just gotten. Delia was sitting, shoes off, in a patient room with maps of Puerto Rico, Saudi Arabia, and Brazil on the walls.

Franco spoke to her in a mix of English and Spanish, asking a hodgepodge of questions: *What kind of things do you like to eat? What's your favorite subject in school? Who is your best friend? Why won't you wear your glasses?*

For almost twenty minutes, Franco conducted a completely average checkup. Ears were clear. Throat looked good, reflexes perfect. She learned that Delia still liked dolls, hadn't started her period yet, wouldn't wear her glasses because her friend told her they looked ugly, and didn't yet know how to ride a bike. Finally, Delia's mother said something Franco found odd—one of the girl's prepubescent breasts hurt.

"How often does that happen?" she asked, suddenly concerned. "It may be a normal part of breast development. I'll check." When she examined the girl's chest, she noticed that the left nipple looked different. It had what seemed like a vein running through it. The nipple hurt when she touched it.

Franco excused herself from the room and sat down at a computer in the hallway. She took a sip of her soy coffee drink and looked up

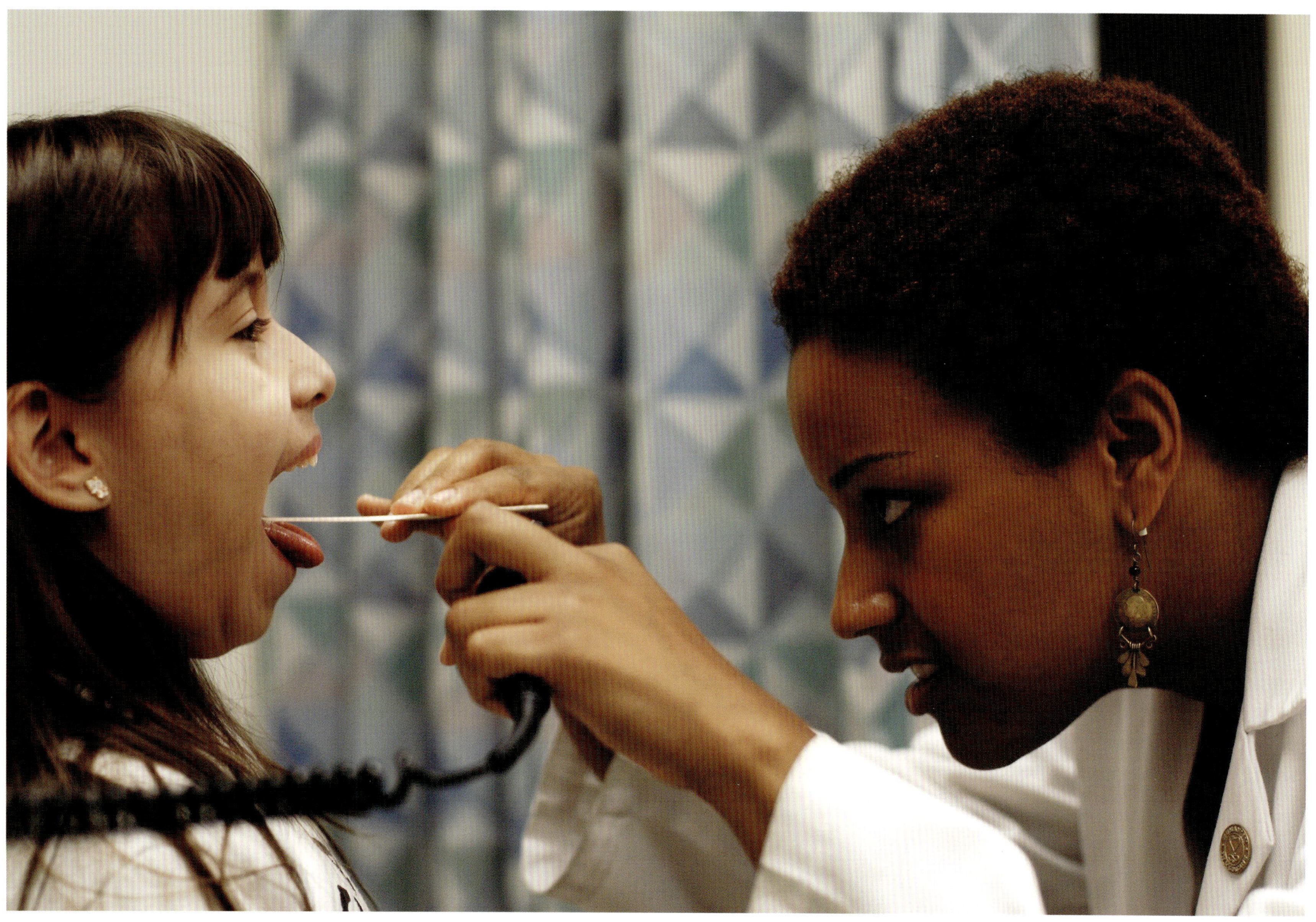

In June 2007, Franco gives ten-year-old Delia a checkup at the Thomas F. McCafferty Health Center on Cleveland's Near West Side.

the Tanner stages of sexual development. Dr. Wendy Cicek greeted her from the phone across the hall. She was on hold with an insurance company from which she was trying to get a preauthorization. This was good use of physician time, she said sarcastically.

Doctors at McCafferty, a center affiliated with MetroHealth Medical Center on Cleveland's West Side, do a lot of this. Many of their patients are Hispanics, who are more than 14 percent less likely than whites to seek and receive health-care coverage, which may be why they have poorer health and higher rates of serious disability and death, according to the Centers for Disease Control and Prevention. Cultural barriers often get in the way, as do language problems. Many McCafferty patients, patients who don't speak English or know their way around the insurance system, need more than doctors. They need doctor-advocates.

That's one reason Franco loved it here. Of all the clinical experiences she'd had, this was the one that most fit her ideal: McCafferty served a poor population—*her* population, or the population she'd belonged to while growing up in Boston's Jamaica Plain neighborhood in the 1990s. The doctors were good there, but they didn't speak Spanish well. Soon Franco became the spokesperson for her family's health. At McCafferty, most doctors did speak Spanish, and the cultural disconnects seemed to be much fewer than she'd experienced in the Boston clinic. Once patients realized she was Dominican, they opened up about all their home remedies. When a patient told her he used Vicks VapoRub for everything, it didn't surprise her. Members of her family had done the same thing.

Franco wrote notes from her visit and her research on a note card, which she held like a security blanket in front of Dr. Douglas Van Auken, the medical director. She stood up straight, preparing to give her presentation. The basic format went through her mind: history of present illness goes first, but checkups are harder because there is no present illness, so she'd just start with telling him it was a checkup. She swallowed hard. She tried not to stutter. Van Auken listened, most of the time without making eye contact.

"She has no issues whatsoever," Franco said in closing. "Just breast tenderness."

No medical issues, but Van Auken continued to bring up new subjects that could affect her well-being. What activities was she in? Was she reading much?

"It's important to talk to her about strangers," he added. "Two girls about her age disappeared around here." He was referring to Amanda Berry and Gina DeJesus, West Side girls who disappeared in 2003 and 2004, respectively. Neither had been found. Franco didn't know that. She added abduction to the long list of things to bring up with this patient population, these younger versions of herself.

Later, in the patient room, Van Auken retraced all of Franco's steps. He allayed the mother's fears about the breast soreness. Before he let them leave, he told Delia to be aware of her surroundings when she's outside. "If someone talks to you on a busy street, what do you do?" he asked.

"Run!" Delia answered.

"Good. What else?"

"Scream!"

"That's exactly right."

I saw Franco one more time that summer, for about fifteen minutes at her apartment, just so I could meet her mom. After that, I couldn't get her on the phone for about four months. I worried I'd offended her somehow in my story about the med students' second year, but Franco wasn't getting back to a lot of people. In fact—and I didn't learn this until months later—she was barely leaving her couch. She

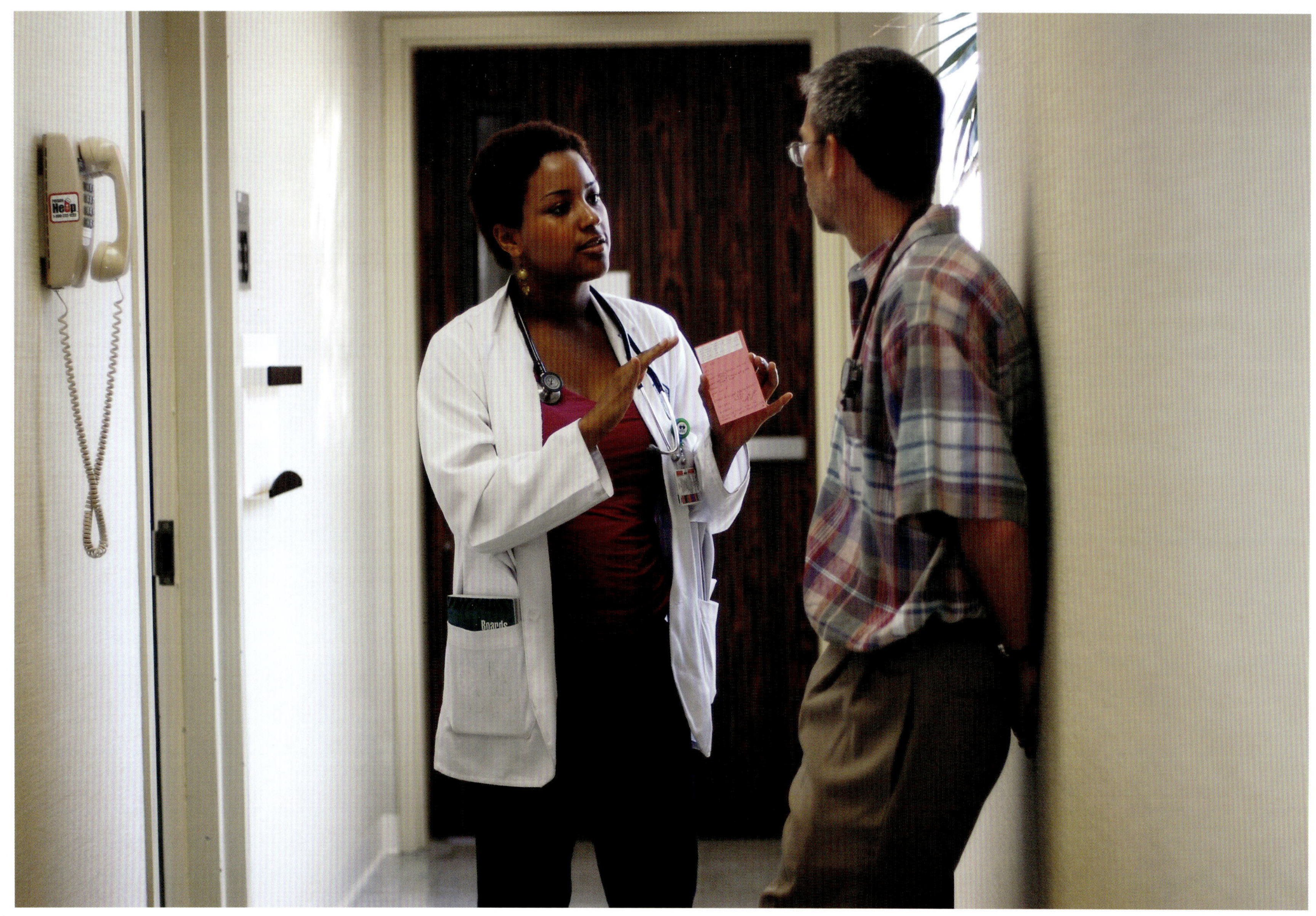

Franco presents her patient report to Dr. Douglas Van Auken. During her third year, she often got nervous when she had to make presentations to the physicians evaluating her.

was exhausted from an incredibly tough first clinical block where she rushed from service to service without ever spending enough time anywhere to feel acclimated. Then days on the couch turned into weeks on the couch. She cried at every little thing. Her mother visited in August, and that cheered her up. But when she left, Franco started crying again. She left her apartment only to get groceries. Once in a while, her boyfriend, a salsa instructor, got her to salsa night at the downtown nightclub View. She never stayed long.

According to a 2005 *New England Journal of Medicine* report, medical students are most at risk of depression during the third and fourth years, when they are separated from their peers and frequently moved into new situations with unfamiliar physicians. Often these experiences are the students' first encounters with illness and death and "may unmask psychological vulnerabilities."

Even though student doctors can often diagnose depression in others, many don't seek treatment themselves. Like Franco, who even hid her symptoms from her friends and family, they fear a depression diagnosis might limit their career opportunities. One study shows that residency directors are less likely to ask a candidate to interview if he or she has a history of counseling, the *New England Journal of Medicine* has pointed out.

Franco was supposed to spend the summer interviewing low-income women about the human papillomavirus vaccine. Instead, she spent it watching daytime television. In September, people at the school contacted her friends, who contacted her family. The phone tree of concern helped her snap out of her funk, as did the realization that she was risking her future.

We finally talked about this in early January 2008, over Dominican food on the Near West Side. It was a snowy day, and the restaurant wasn't as crowded as I would have liked. In our conversation, Franco was unusually cautious. Her natural inclination toward honesty about her medical school experiences seemed in conflict with her desire not to imperil her chances at getting a good residency. She'd read the research on depression in medical school. She didn't care how common it is. If she was completely open about her condition, it could be one more thing holding her back.

I asked her for specifics: *What happened exactly? When did you go from feeling normal to being couch-bound? When did you decide you would try to get better?* Franco, usually a natural at cataloging both the minor details and the major epiphanies of her life, was still trying to figure out the answers to these questions herself. She suspected the idleness of the research block contributed to her problem, and she decided against taking more time off from school. She changed the order of her coursework, doing her electives first and delaying the research block. She started seeing a counselor.

One doctor who'd become depressed in med school warned Franco about the psych rotation, but she was eager to do it anyway. She ended up seeing so many professionals, so many "normal" people with "normal" lives, that it actually made her feel better about her own depressive episode. Psychiatric diseases, she quickly learned, don't discriminate.

At the end of that rotation, Franco found herself standing before the attending physician in psychiatry at University Hospitals Case Medical Center, wanting to disagree with him. It had been seven months since she got pricked by a contaminated scalpel in the OR and one month since she learned she was negative for both HIV and hepatitis C. (The rapid HIV test came back in an hour, but she had to wait six months for the results of the hepatitis C test.)

Her vertigo was better, and she hardly resembled the nervous third-year student she'd been, the one afraid to open her mouth in front of attending physicians. It helped that psychiatry was one of her favorite rotations. Although it was not the McCafferty clinic—there were no cute kids getting checkups, no easy rapport with other native Spanish speakers—the inpatient psych ward was interesting and unpredictable. She was talking with a patient eating orange slices one minute and cleaning them off her shoes—after the patient hurled them at her—the next.

The psych team asked her opinion on every patient. Most of the time she agreed with the attending physician, but not in the case of a normally high-functioning bipolar woman. He wanted her released. Was he sure, Franco asked, given the woman's obviously speeded-up speech pattern? Franco was glad she mustered the confidence to challenge him, even if he didn't end up agreeing with her. As if on cue, the patient Franco wanted to keep in the hospital started talking really fast, as if someone had pressed the fast-forward button. After witnessing this, the attending decided Franco was right about the patient acting too manic to be released.

At the end of the rotation, he asked Franco if she'd consider becoming a psychiatrist.

•◆◆◆•

In June 2007, four months after beginning his third year in medical school, Mike Norton was sworn into the U.S. Army Reserve as a second lieutenant. Norton's family planned to fly in for the ceremony, but they ended up missing it because Norton got commissioned a week early by a two-star general who happened to be in town. I joined Nor-

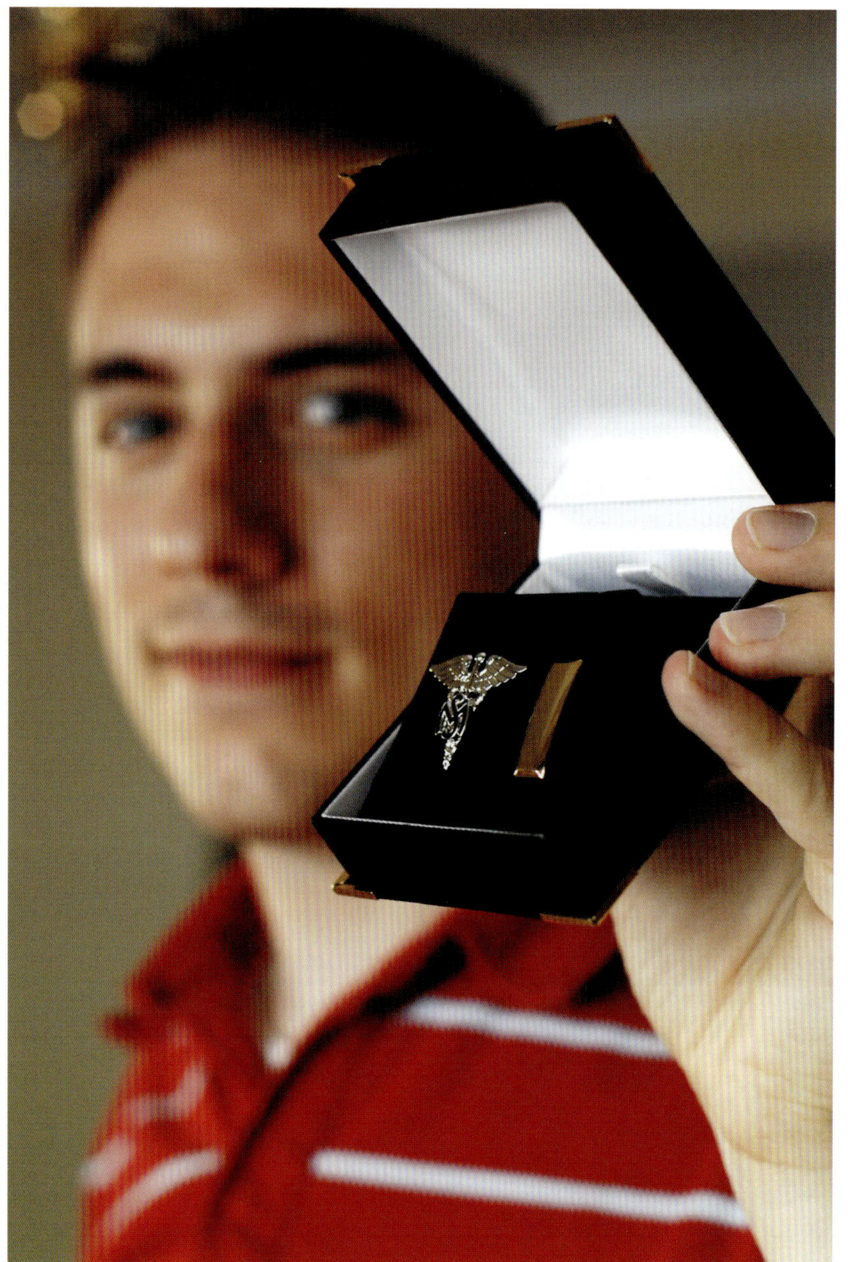

Soon after being commissioned into the U.S. Army Reserve in June 2007, Norton receives this insignia for the Medical Services Corps, as well as the single gold bar of the second lieutenant.

ton's parents at his house soon after they arrived. When I got there, they were trimming shrubs and doing other work around the rental property. Toni, Norton's mom, told me stories while she played with Megan, her first grandchild, who had grown from a warm, blonde bundle into an energetic toddler with just enough hair for pigtail sprouts. Norton's father shook my hand and smiled warmly.

Bryan Norton didn't know this at the time, but his son and daughter-in-law were planning to name their next child, a boy, after him. Robert Bryan Norton II was due in November 2007. "I want Robby to go through life with that name and have that to live up to," Norton told me.

Robby was early, born October 22, 2007, and Norton took three days off from his family medicine rotation to get to know him. I didn't make it to the hospital to witness this Norton birth, unfortunately. The amount of time I could spend following the students had decreased significantly in their third year for several reasons. I had left the magazine for a tenure-track job at Kent State University, where I taught journalism. In my second year, I was still getting used to teaching three classes—most of them writing intensive—per semester while handling all the other service and research obligations of the position. I was also five months pregnant with a baby girl due in March 2008. In addition to my personal circumstances, getting access to the wards, where the students spent most of their time, proved to be more difficult than popping by the students' classes, as I had done during the first two years. To secure permission to shadow them in the hospitals, the students and I had to go through several layers of gatekeepers, including hospital public-relations staffers, attending physicians, and, of course, patients.

I didn't visit the Nortons until two weeks after Robby's birth. He was sleeping in his swing and wearing a yellow sleeper that said, "He's not just my daddy . . . he's my hero." Norton asked if I wanted to hold him, but I said no. I didn't want to disturb him. But Norton assured me that moving Robby from his beloved swing to a stranger's arms would not wake him up.

Norton still hadn't settled on a specialty. He said Dr. Walsh was the toughest instructor he'd ever had. Although his strategies for teaching seemed too harsh for some medical students, Norton found them effective. He sometimes stayed late—even breaking the rule that med students should spend no more than eighty hours a week in the hospital—to watch more of Walsh's surgeries.

"What do you think I don't like about this note," he once asked Norton, who had no idea what the problem could be with a patient note he had written.

"It's verbose?"

"It's too clean," Walsh replied. "It's too messy of a situation for this note."

The surgeon advised him to stop looking for a clean clinical picture, the kind Norton could always figure out on exams. Real people are more complex; they have a variety of ailments. Sometimes they don't tell you what you need to know; sometimes they lie.

Norton felt a lot like J. D. on his favorite sitcom, *Scrubs,* the likeable goof who's always trying to win the approval of his mentor, Dr. Cox, who pretends to detest him as he constantly demeans him. (Cox tells J. D. in one episode: "It was me who saw you doing leg lifts in the gym on that inflatable ball. It was quite the display of girl power.") Even though Walsh never questioned his gender identification or called him "Lassie," Norton was still worried about what the surgeon thought of him. Throughout the surgery rotation, Norton's feelings of inadequacy were heightened anytime he had one of his frequent ADHD-prompted "foot-in-mouth" episodes.

In Walsh's evaluation, however, Norton found the affirmation he had been seeking in person for so long. "Norton is a hardworking, compulsive individual who constantly works hard to excel," Walsh wrote. "He is bright and has a very good fund of knowledge. . . . Overall, his performance has been quite good and he may consider a career in surgery."

Walsh believed in him, even as he understood something important about him. Norton *was* compulsive—it could be his biggest problem. Yet Walsh did not think it would keep him from becoming a surgeon. Norton's marriage, however, was another story.

It's 7 P.M. when third-year medical student Mike Norton throws his coat into a heap behind the nurses' station at MacDonald Women's Hospital. He wears clean scrubs, but his shoes still have umbilical cord blood on them from the night before.

An amplified fetal heartbeat pounds out of a nearby room. He knows the heartbeat can speed up—*knockknockknock*—or slow down—*knock . . . knock . . . knock*—causing flutters of activity and flurries of emotion. Sometimes it just pads along like a ticking clock he forgets is there. *Knock, knock, knock.*

They lost a baby on the floor the week before Norton arrived. A walkway connects MacDonald to Rainbow Babies and Children's Hospital, and most babies born here do fine. Still, this is a city hospital. In one room, a teenager in her second trimester is having labor pains, and she's had no prenatal care. In another, a fifteen-year-old labors actively, her pregnant eighteen-year-old sister and her thirty-something mother waiting nearby.

At 7:15, Norton visits Ramiasha Muhammad. She's contracting every two to five minutes. He asks if she'd be comfortable with his doing a cervical exam. She says yes. After twelve hours of labor, she's six centimeters dilated. Four more to go before she can start pushing.

After that exam, he sits in a room no one is using, waiting for something to do.

Norton sees younger versions of himself waiting all over this floor: in the hallway, the first-year medical student waits for a doctor who never shows. In Room 6, the nervous first-time expectant father waits for a whole day to meet his daughter, Megan. In Room 8, the nervous second-time expectant father waits for his son, Robby, to be born.

Across the hall, someone pushes a swollen and crying postpartum woman in a wheelchair. Labor and delivery is a place of miracles and nightmares. So far, he's been lucky.

He's seen only miracles.

At 1:17 A.M., Ramiasha's room fills with doctors and nurses. The baby's heart rate is dropping. Gloves are pulled on, masks placed, scrubs draped.

"You're having a contraction," a doctor tells Ramiasha. "Take a deep breath and push."

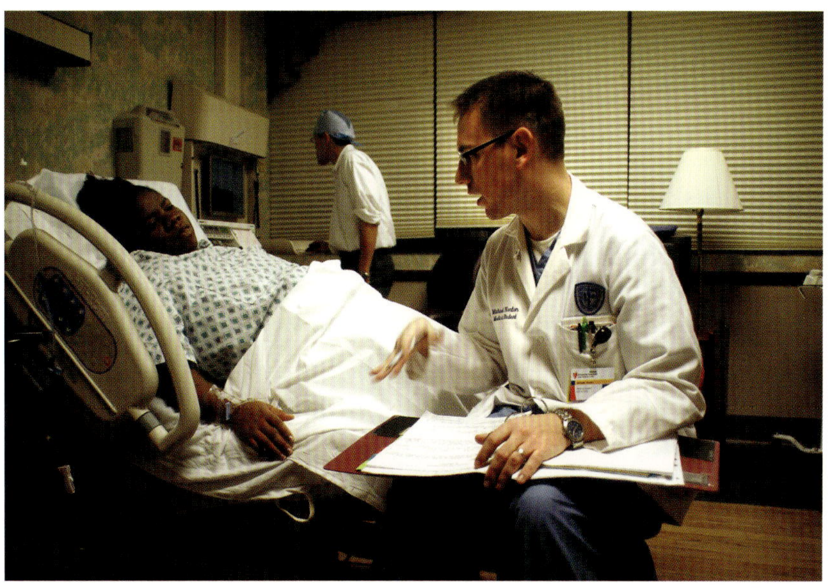

Norton spent more time on the labor and delivery floor than most medical students did—his wife had two babies there in three years. This was the clinical setting where I saw him the most. On November 28, 2007, he visits with Ramiasha Muhammad, who is in labor.

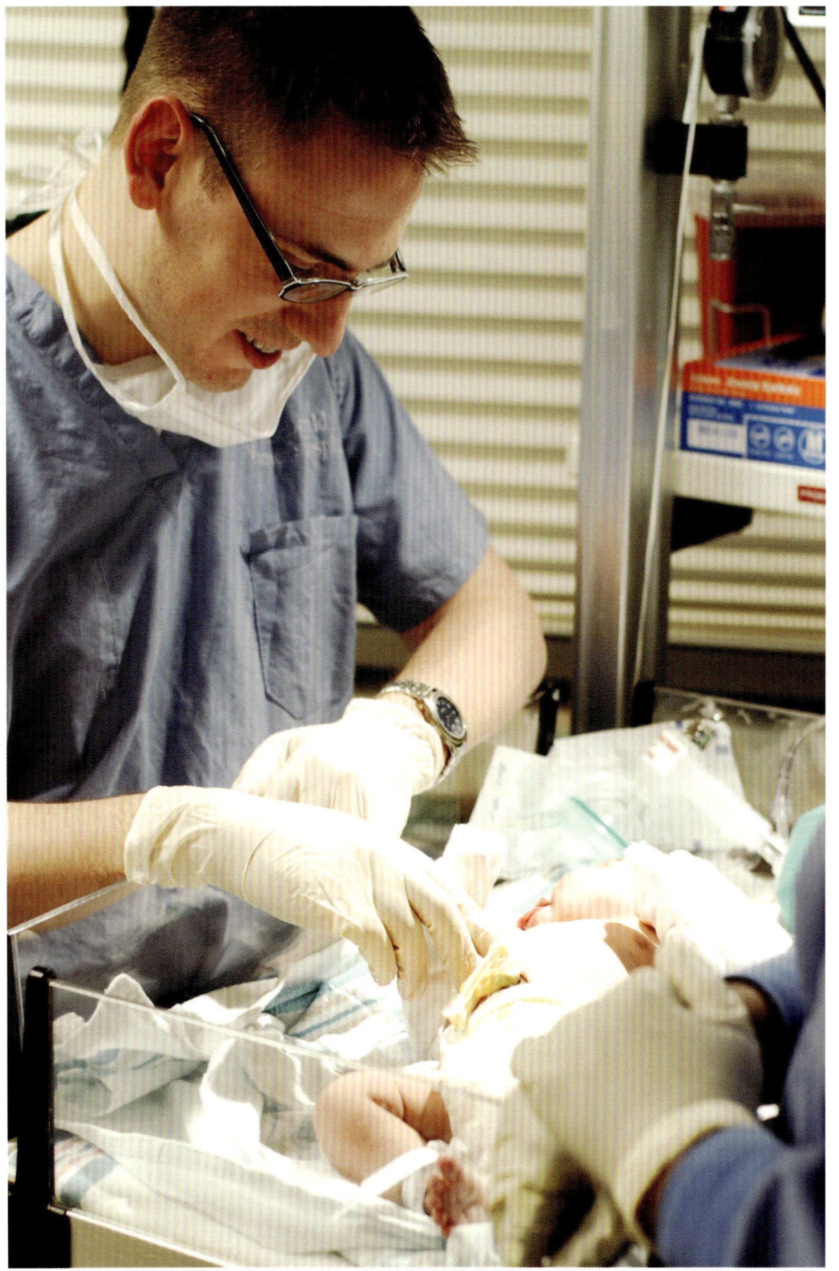

"Push, push, push," a nurse says.

The baby's heartbeat thumps out of the monitor, *knock, knock, knock.*

"Push, push, push. One . . . two . . . three . . . four . . . five . . . six . . . seven . . . eight . . . nine . . . ten."

Knock, knock, knock, knockknockknockknockknock.

"Push!"

The head emerges, waxy and curly-haired.

At 1:31 A.M., the baby cries. "She's got lungs," the doctor says. Loud, beautiful lungs.

Norton delivers the placenta and slops the dark red blob in a metal basin. He sidesteps the huge bag of blood under the delivery table.

"That's why these are my hospital shoes," he says.

He doesn't care if he gets more blood on them. It's another miracle.

Norton was excited to help a new mother give birth, even though he just got to deliver the placenta. Here, he checks the baby girl's vitals.

The Specialties

So I am in the emergency department today like I am every freaking day. I hear all the residents' and attending physicians' pagers go off at the same time, which means there's a trauma victim en route. A minute later, the announcement is made (in case you didn't get the page), "A doctor, a nurse, and a medic needed in Trauma Bay 11. ETA five minutes." Usually, I rush over to the traumas, but I was busy trying to get a line in a patient who desperately needed fluids, so I take my time.

When I walk over to the trauma bay to observe, I see that there are plenty of people there. My senior resident says, "Put on some gloves." I put them on. The patient arrives. This 96-year-old little old lady, already intubated. While someone is bagging her—blowing air through a tube into her lungs—and someone else is doing chest compressions, I watch because this is actually the first medical resuscitation I've ever witnessed.

We get the story from the paramedic: The patient was found by her family. She was without a pulse for over 30 minutes. They had given her all sorts of meds to jumpstart her heart, then she got shocked (like they do in the movies), but nothing, so they brought her to us.

Then my senior resident says to me, "Would you need the step?" And I look at her like she's crazy because I have no idea what she's talking about. Then she points to this movable step that's next to me. "You want to make sure you're standing over the patient," she says, "because you're kind of short. You would need the step to do chest compressions." And I nod because I think she's bringing this up in a hypothetical way, like, "Marleny, if you ever needed to do compressions, you would need the step." So, I say, "Yeah, I would need the step." Then she says, "Good, then carry it in and take over." What is going through my mind is "Ummm, did I ever mention that, while I have read about chest compressions, I have not actually done them?" But I didn't say anything because, well, I just didn't think that's something she wanted to hear, not to mention that if I did them wrong, surely people would correct me and take over.

So, I take the step and stand over this lady who has no pulse, and I start doing compressions. All of a sudden, I hear a man (the attending physician) say to me, "Faster! Deeper! Harder!" And I'm like, "Oh, OK." So I go faster, deeper, harder. He says, "If you're doing it right, you should be sweating, your muscles should be burning! Your goal is at least 100 compressions per minute." And my muscles are burning! That shit hurts!

Anyway, it is a really sad, humbling, and strangely thrilling experience. I just keep thinking, Wow, we may actually be able to bring this woman back. But we don't. I mean, she had little to no chance, having been without a pulse for 30 minutes before paramedics got there. But for a split second, I think just how cool it would be if we bring her back, and if I have a role in it.

Afterwards, my attending pulls me to the side and says, "Good job. Did you break any of her ribs?" I say, "No. I didn't feel any break." He says, "Yeah, I think the big medic who was doing compressions before you probably did. Well, even if you had, just remember that's not what matters. You have to go hard and deep and fast if you want a chance at saving someone's life. So don't let the possibility of broken ribs deter you from doing what you need to do."

What a day.

In this post for her blog, Franco described what it was like—finally—to perform a medical act that could save a life. Only after standing on that moveable step doing those chest compressions faster, deeper, harder did she realize that she could not have saved *that* life. It might not be too late, however, for her next patient. After this experience, Franco knew the right way to do chest compressions. Hard, deep, and fast. You can't worry about breaking ribs.

Franco was in the right place at the right time, but she was also looking for that experience. Medical knowledge isn't worth anything if you can't put it to good use. By year 4, students know that. That's when they do advanced work in the clinical specialties, and they get more opportunities like this one in the emergency department. They ask themselves the questions that will help them decide on their future specialties: Do I want to treat children? Do I want to do surgery? Do I want to be on the cutting edge of research? Do I want to see the same patients over and over? Do I want to make a lot of money? Am I willing to sacrifice money for more flexible hours? The questions often lead to more questions. No medical specialty custom fits anyone's life, but you don't want to squeeze into a size 4 if you're a 10.

By her fourth year, Gentry knew radiology was the right choice. Dermatology was even more competitive, and she knew she'd never make it as a pediatrician. Ultimately, it wasn't the bad hours and relatively low pay that turned her off to the field. She loved kids, but she discovered it was hard for her to see them really sick. In one outpatient clinic, she saw a nine-year-old boy who was sexually abusing his sister, doing to her what had been done to him by his drug-addicted parents, and she couldn't get him out of her mind. As a pediatrician, "I'd be worrying about these kids all the time," she said.

During fourth year, she enjoyed hearing from peers who had changed their minds about the sort of doctor they wanted to be. Even if they'd once wanted to pursue illustrious careers in surgery, look for the cure for cancer, or spend their days treating sick children in the Third World, some were choosing less personally demanding specialties, such as radiology and anesthesiology. They wanted to wear the long white coat, but they wanted to wear some other garments too: an apron, perhaps, or a jogging suit or an evening gown. They wanted fulfilling jobs, along with families and travel and pagers they would be able to turn off sometimes.

Residency was approaching, and the students had to decide where they wanted to spend the next few years of their lives. All three struggled to write personal statements. These narratives had to reflect their growth, dedication, and future plans—and hit all the right notes residency directors like to hear.

In her first year, Franco marveled at the ease with which patients and their parents talked to the pediatrician she shadowed, Dr. Mark Feingold, and at his ability to be both straightforward and reassuring. In three hours, she never saw him take a break. He displayed the kind of empathy, diligence, and connection to patients that she wanted to have someday. His urban hospital, MetroHealth, was the sort of place where Franco could envision working. Known for its LifeFlight helicopter rescues and its excellent burn center, Metro-

Health also treats very sick, very poor patients. The one Franco remembered most clearly from that day, however, the baby of a teenage single mother, was not the sort of patient Franco would like to see regularly. She was too healthy.

In college, Franco had worked with seriously ill children at a summer camp in Connecticut. There, she'd found she didn't get overly saddened by very sick kids, like some people do. She'd seen the happiness on a wheelchair-bound kid's face when he climbed into a hot-air balloon, and there's nothing like it. More than keeping healthy kids healthy, she liked to help sick kids feel normal. So she was considering a pediatric specialty. Although she regretted not completing her research on time because of her depression, it did give her one advantage: she took her electives, which were part of the fourth-year curriculum, early. She completed one in pediatric gastrointestinal medicine and another in adolescent medicine. Both reaffirmed her desire to work with sick kids—a diverse population of sick kids.

"I want to work in the inner city," she told me. "I feel it's my duty. If I'm not going to do it and I come from there, then who's going to do it? And I want to do it."

In her personal statement, she described a trip she'd taken to the pediatrician's office when she was nine and new to the United States. The doctor got "an incomplete history using hand gestures and single-word sentences: '*Vacunas?*' (Immunizations?) '*Dolor?*' (Pain?) '*Fiebre?*' (Fever?)" Those encounters made her mother feel as powerless as her children. As a teenager, Franco realized how language and cultural barriers lead to worse health outcomes. "I realized that I was surrounded by living proof in my neighborhood. There was our elderly neighbor who, in order to avoid the hassle of a medical interview in English, preferred to treat her chronic cough with other people's antibiotics. Down the street, there was the asthmatic child who, unbeknownst to his physician, was being treated with herbal teas and syrups instead of inhaled corticosteroids. As one would expect, both experienced significant morbidity."

Franco wanted to help people like her former neighbors. Even in med school, she'd sought out volunteer and research opportunities focused on reducing health-care disparities. But, ultimately, she decided she also wanted to see a variety of children across the economic spectrum. In her personal statement, she said she knew she wanted to do this because of Jay, an eleven-year-old boy with persistent severe asthma.

> I met Jay in the emergency department, where he was seeking treatment for yet another asthma exacerbation. My attending, a pulmonologist, and I had been called in for a consult. Jay sat on the side of the bed with a nebulizer mouthpiece in his mouth. His mother, sitting beside him, began to recount her attempts to manage his symptoms at home. After examining him, we decided to admit him to the floor for scheduled albuterol treatments.
>
> Several hours later, we checked in on Jay only to find him more fatigued, now with diffuse wheezing and increased retractions. Jay needed continuous albuterol treatments, so I went to find a nurse to administer it. Upon my return ten minutes later, Jay was hunched over, appearing ashen, with sunken eyes. My attending and I placed our stethoscopes on his back and, in concert, shot one another looks of concern: Jay's previously noisy lungs had grown quieter due to decreased air exchange. As my attending arranged transport to the PICU, Jay

began to vomit. He was agitated, crying and retching. I could see the panic in his eyes. As nurses ran in and out of the room with buckets and towels, I stayed with Jay, rubbing his back and wiping the sweat off his forehead.

When Jay stopped crying and vomiting, I realized that his mother was no longer by his side. She was standing behind the curtain by the window, out of Jay's sight. As I approached her, she softly sobbed. Between sobs, she said, "I just feel so helpless, like I can't do anything for him." At that moment, she reminded me of my mother. Jay's mother is not an immigrant. There was no cultural or language barrier. But at that moment, she felt powerless and scared, just as my mother felt when I was nine. I put my arm around her, searching for words to reassure her. I finally said, "Together, we'll take good care of Jay. You can help now by holding his hand."

Franco wrote about how this experience helped her learn something important. Her mother's powerlessness stemmed from language and cultural barriers in the health-care system. But all parents—even the light-skinned native English speakers among them—feel vulnerable when their children are seriously ill. The suffering of one group doesn't trump that of another. Rich or poor, pain is pain. Everyone needs a doctor to be able and compassionate. Finally, after four years in medical school, she felt she could be that physician.

• ◆ • ◆ •

I expected Gentry to have a harder time with the personal statement. She hates to act the way others want her to act. "I'm a terrible faker," she told me on more than one occasion. "I cannot kiss ass." She still thinks this quality led to her biggest struggles in med school, but in the fourth year, she and Case Med seemed to reach a detente. During her electives, she found out she was great at placing IV's and intubating patients. She even placed an A-line—a tube that goes right into an artery—on her first try.

Gentry mentored first-year students in physical diagnosis, teaching them how to interview patients and take blood pressures. She volunteered at the Free Medical Clinic of Greater Cleveland, where she helped treat patients who had no insurance. She even took on a teaching role at the school. On the morning of September 10, 2008, I watched her run a small group of second-year students in a brightly lit study room with cinderblock walls, marker boards, metal chairs, and no windows. The students rifled through thick textbooks and tapped notes on their laptops. I didn't see any Facebook pages up.

Some students were dressed in ties and skirts, but Gentry, like a few others, wore jeans. She led the group through an "I.Q. Case," a clinical problem developed by faculty members. One by Dr. Robert Bonomo was called "Elena Goodman, Bacterial Endocarditis." The goal: "Students will describe the diagnostic, therapeutic, and medical/surgical management of a blood stream infection." Gentry was supposed to facilitate the students' thinking process, making sure they completed all the learning objectives. There were nine, beginning with "Describe the risk factors, pathophysiology and the protean clinical manifestations of endocarditis." She needed to be there if they had questions, but she was supposed to let them find their own way.

During her first year, these students didn't spend long days in the lecture hall like Gentry had. They still went to the lecture hall, one student told me, only what happened there was no longer called lecture. "It's an interactive large-group experience," she said. Much of

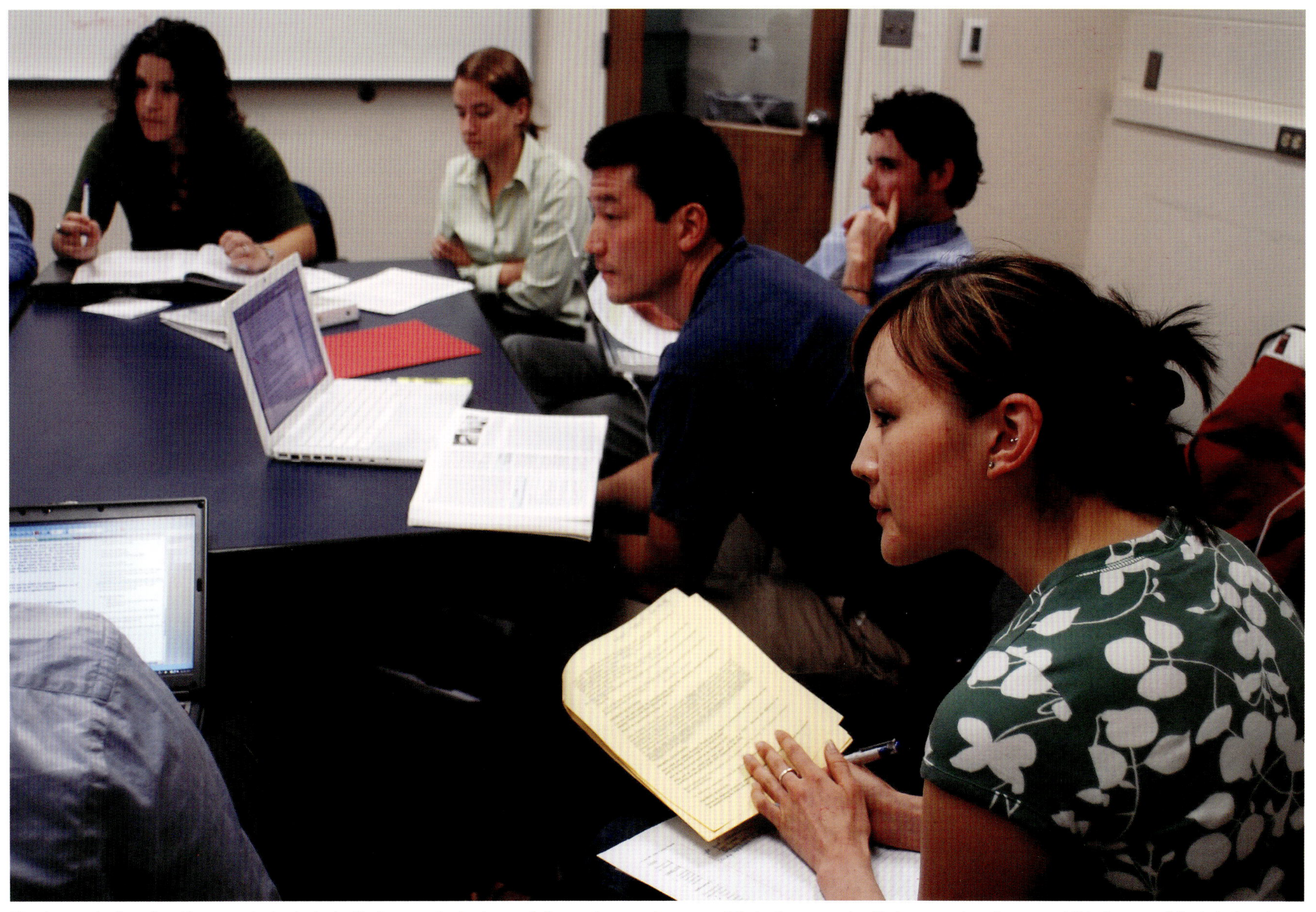

Gentry and other fourth-year students help first-year students work through sample cases. All doctors eventually become teachers, and this is one of their baby steps.

their instruction, however, was conducted in small groups where the students were responsible for teaching themselves.

The students seemed to like her, and she liked them. But she was getting ready to quit everything she didn't have to do to graduate. Two weeks earlier, her mother had been diagnosed with a tumor—a two-and-a-half-inch meningioma outside her brain. She'd had emergency surgery. The neurosurgeon assured them he'd gotten the tumor out. But the recovery had been slow, Gentry told me. Her mother still had a great deal of swelling. She was dizzy, her ear hurt, and she wasn't "all there."

Gentry flew home to help. She took her mother to a follow-up appointment with a neurosurgeon and got enraged. "He was so rude," Gentry recalled. "He didn't answer [my mother's] questions. Mom was dizzy, falling down, and he said it's not his issue." The same went for the problems she had with her medication. Not his problem. Talk to the neurologist.

That was when Gentry got angry. Her mother deserved better than this. Her first day in medical school she would have treated her mother better than this.

"When I started medical school, I was really excited thinking about how we were going to learn to do great things, camaraderie, learn great stuff, and that absolutely didn't happen at all," she told me soon after this experience. "Doctors really don't get any of the support they need anymore. What we do has made us really bitter because nobody appreciates us. . . . We get treated really poorly as students, and people assume we're going to have great and wonderful rides. We miss a lot of years. We take on a lot of debt. We have to delay so many things in our life." In the midst of all this, she had to write that personal statement for residency. I asked her to send what she had so far. She didn't think all of it was very good.

Gentry's narrative was less personal than Franco's. There were no epiphanies, no kids. Since Gentry was not an experienced ass-kisser, it was obvious she was trying to impress with sentences such as this: "I am excited to enter a field that will challenge me to defy convention and to create tools and methods that will allow us to further transform the face of medicine." But other parts of her statement-in-progress sounded like her. She noted her passion for improving women's health, something prompted perhaps by her experience growing up in a rural area with limited access to health care. She valued "creativity and innovation, and radiology is a discipline that combines both."

> A successful radiologist must think outside the box to take a nebulous black and white image and use nothing but his or her eyes and intellect to interpret this picture. Then, he or she must construct a narrative that not only describes the image before them, but also relays a message that can be used to understand the anatomy and pathophysiology of the patient to determine a diagnosis and a successful treatment plan. This is far from easy, and it requires a deep understanding of normal anatomy and the ability to determine what minor and major deviations from the norm are meaningful.
>
> I have spent a great deal of my life teaching, working with a diverse array of students, from toddlers to medical students. These experiences have shown me that I love sharing my knowledge and passions to help students develop their own strengths and interests. As well, the mentorship and teaching and guidance I have received have been invaluable, and I would not be ready to enter a field I know I will love without the help and support of the physicians I have been so fortunate

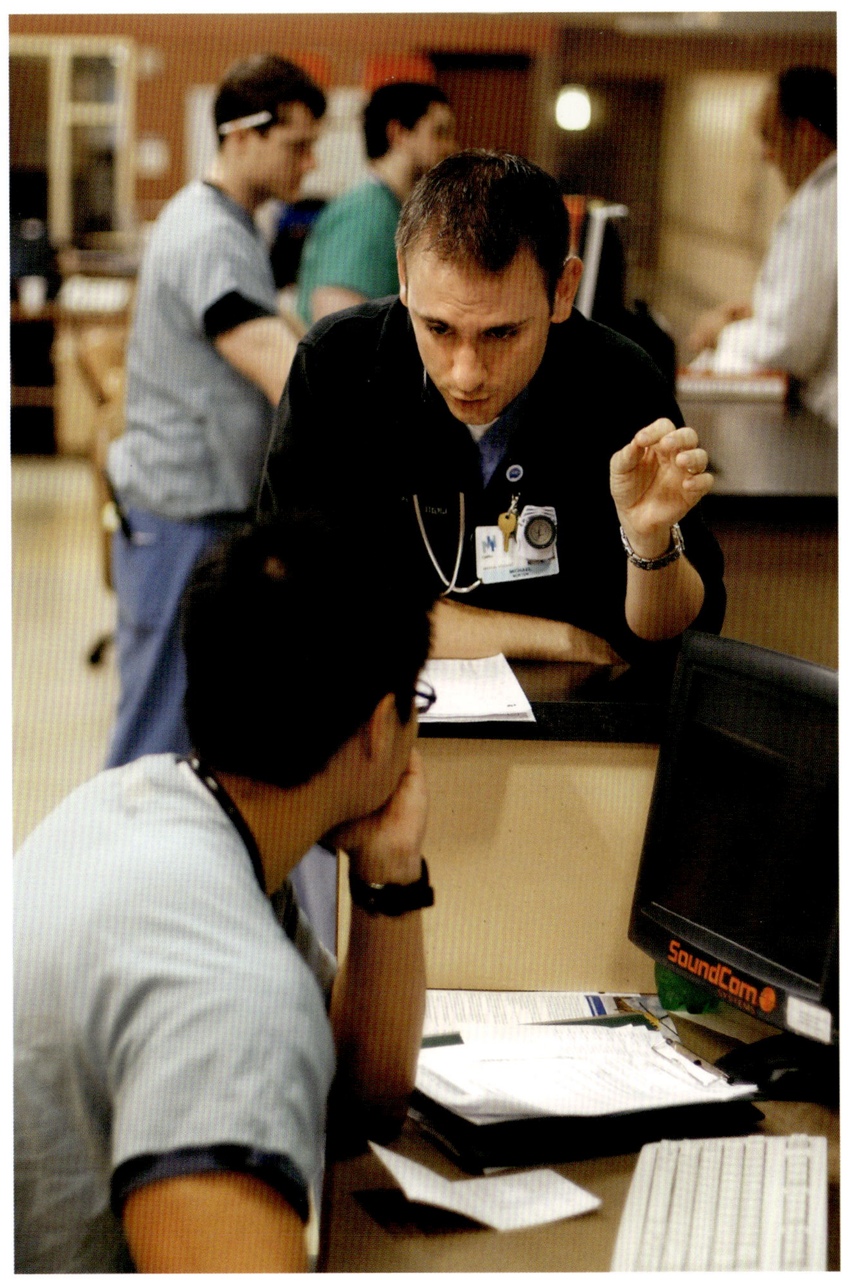

to work with. I am excited to serve as a mentor and role model to a new generation of medical students.

She gave the statement to one of the doctors she worked with. He told her it was really good, but it didn't matter. They may not even read it.

•◆◆◆•

For much of Norton's third year in medical school, Kate cried whenever she thought about her husband becoming a surgeon. She knew he could do the work—he had both the mind and the hands for it.

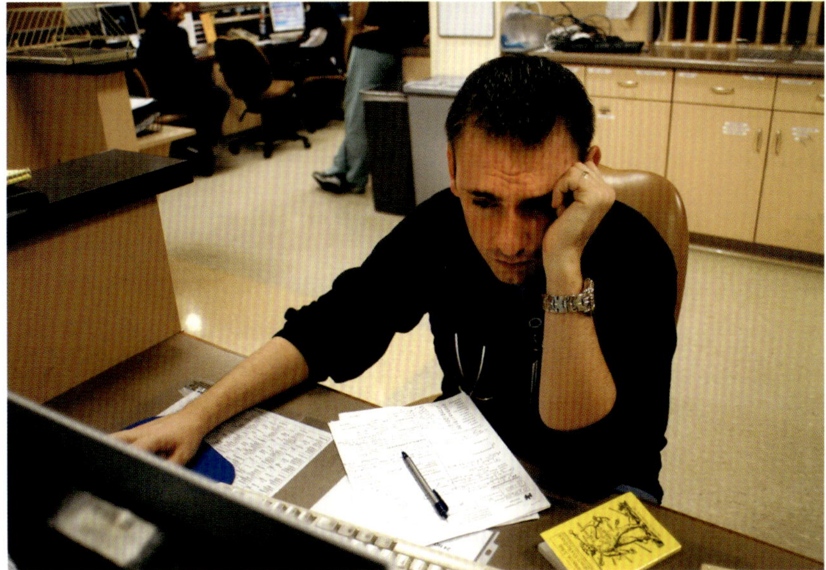

In November 2008, Norton does a rotation in the emergency department of MetroHealth Medical Center. It's here that he sees someone die for the first time. While medical students often witness the deaths of patients, the gravity of Norton's experience was compounded by the knowledge that he would soon be on the other side of the curtain. At the time, his father was in the late stages of ALS.

During Bridge Week, the week before the beginning of the third year on the wards, I watched the students learn to suture and tie knots on model arms made of rubber. Norton made his first knot on the first try. He repeated it again and again to make sure he wouldn't forget it. Then he spent the rest of the time helping the students sitting around him.

Despite having both the passion for surgery and the hands, Norton liked gold stars, Kate said, and the surgeons he encountered didn't hand them out much. To Kate, those surgeons seemed different from other doctors. They were more competitive, less warm. While he was being "pimped" during one surgery, for instance, Norton gave the wrong answer and the attending corrected him brusquely then demanded he stop talking. This behavior would seem rude anywhere else, but it was acceptable, even expected, in the OR. When Norton came home, he was a wreck, Kate said. "He's not capable of leaving it at the hospital."

During third year, Norton was on edge all the time, worrying about his evaluations, his grades, some stupid thing he'd said that he then stupidly tried to explain. During his surgery rotation, Kate felt she was more therapist than spouse. When Norton was done talking with Kate, he called his father. He talked to Bryan about the latest embarrassment and got his take on things. Bryan always knew everything, from what elective he should take to what was wrong with the car. Just hearing his voice calmed Norton down.

By third year, Kate was used to spending little time with her husband. She was busy with the kids and had developed a good network of student and resident wives. In the Case archives, I found a listing for an organization for medical students' wives. The file had only one sheet in it. It stated that the Medical Students' Wives Association of Western Reserve University "awards the honorable degree of P.H.T., Put Husband Through. To: (add name) for having successfully, meritoriously, and lovingly encouraged, aided her lawful spouse to more comfortable living and higher academic achievements." So all I found out about the organization, if it did actually exist, was that its members had a sense of humor.

Although they weren't an official organization, some wives of medical students in Norton's class did get together. They talked about the same things medical students' wives have probably always talked about—how their husbands were handling things, the children, the future. Kate knew Norton loved surgery, but he was still open to other possibilities—and that gave her hope. During his third-year psychiatry rotation at University Hospitals, an anesthesiology resident whose name really was Jerry Garcia told Norton he'd planned to be a surgeon in medical school, too, until he took an anesthesiology elective. He suggested that Norton do the same. Kate liked what she heard about anesthesia—better hours, good pay, fewer egos, more team-based work—and she encouraged Norton to follow Garcia's lead.

In April of his third year, Norton took an anesthesiology elective at MetroHealth. He got to be part of a four-member anesthesia team that resuscitated a man with a life-threatening post-operative hemorrhage so the surgeons could cut him open again. It was like something out of the movies—the surgeons running down the hall with the stretcher answering questions the anesthesiologists fired at them. Norton was the "go-to boy," getting blood and doing whatever else anyone told him to do. He noticed how the others on the team worked together seamlessly, practically reading one another's minds. This was fun, Norton thought, maybe as fun as surgery, and not as grueling. He recognized that he would have to give up some of the glory—maybe all the glory. That man's family was going to remember the surgeons who stopped the hemorrhaging, not the anesthesiologists who resuscitated him. Like surgery, though, anesthesiology offered plenty of intellectual stimulation, and the lifestyle would afford him more time with his family. Because Norton was in the Army, anesthesiology would also mean less time on active duty—only three years after his residency—to pay the government back for taking on his med school tab. Kate would support him no matter what, but they wanted more kids, and he didn't want her to raise them alone.

After that anesthesiology elective, Norton was more confused than ever. He wasn't ready to give up on surgery and did another surgery rotation at Madigan Army Medical Center in Washington state. The month-long rotation would end with an interview for a residency spot at the hospital, which was in an ideal location, just three hours from Kate's parents' house. After long days in the OR, he came back to his hotel room completely exhausted, to find a bunch of research waiting for him. He called Kate, who was staying with the kids at her parents' place for the month. Over the phone, she heard the indecision in his voice slowly fade. He loved surgery. He couldn't deny that. But he didn't want to be this tired all the time. He canceled his interview for the surgery residency at Madigan.

"A surgeon told me, 'If you could be happy doing something other than surgery, then surgery isn't for you,'" he said. "I could be happy doing something other than surgery."

He decided "something" was definitely anesthesiology. Jerry Garcia changed his life—and that's what he wrote in his residency application.

The Match

Obsessing over her future kept Gentry up at night. When she did sleep, nightmares woke her. Her score for step 1 of the United States Medical Licensing Examination, though in the average range, was relatively low for radiology. She would be competing with students who studied more, dressed snappier, and got less distracted by cookbooks. (By the end of fourth year, she had amassed about seventy.) Many radiologists enjoy regular business hours and a high salary, even by physician standards. In 2009, radiologists were offered an average salary of about $391,000, according to the health-care job search firm Merritt Hawkins & Associates, which compiles such information from the searches it does each year. Compare that to the average pediatrician's offer, which comes with middle-of-the-night calls, at $171,000.

Medical students, especially those trying to get competitive residencies like Gentry, spend their fourth year on the road, interviewing at as many residency programs as possible. Then they compile a list of the programs they like, ranking them in order of preference. The residency programs make their own lists. Applicants and programs are not allowed to request one another's list or ask for a specific ranking. Expressions of interest are fine, but there is no "If you rank me number 1, I'll rank you number 1" allowed. An impartial not-for-profit corporation, the National Resident Matching Program, processes the lists and spits out the matches. Its placements are binding. The process is supposed to protect both parties from making decisions before they know all their options, but it is sheer torture for medical students.

Norton and the other fourth-year students in the armed forces got to skip much of this drama. They competed for spots at military hospitals and only got to join the regular matching program if a match could not be found in their specialties. Norton ranked Brooke Army Medical Center in San Antonio number 1 because of the anesthesia experience he would be likely to get there—and because it was the farthest west he could get. The Army website said the match would be posted in December—three months before civilian medical students found out where they matched. He and Kate signed on at 6 A.M. that day. When they saw he'd gotten his first choice, they went back to bed because it would be several hours before their families on the West Coast awoke.

Franco, Gentry, and the other students didn't submit their final lists until the end of February. Then they waited three weeks for Black Monday, the day med students find out *if* they have been matched to a program. "People become doctors because they want to have a sense of security," Gentry said. "You lose all of that with the residency match." Every year, there are medical students who don't

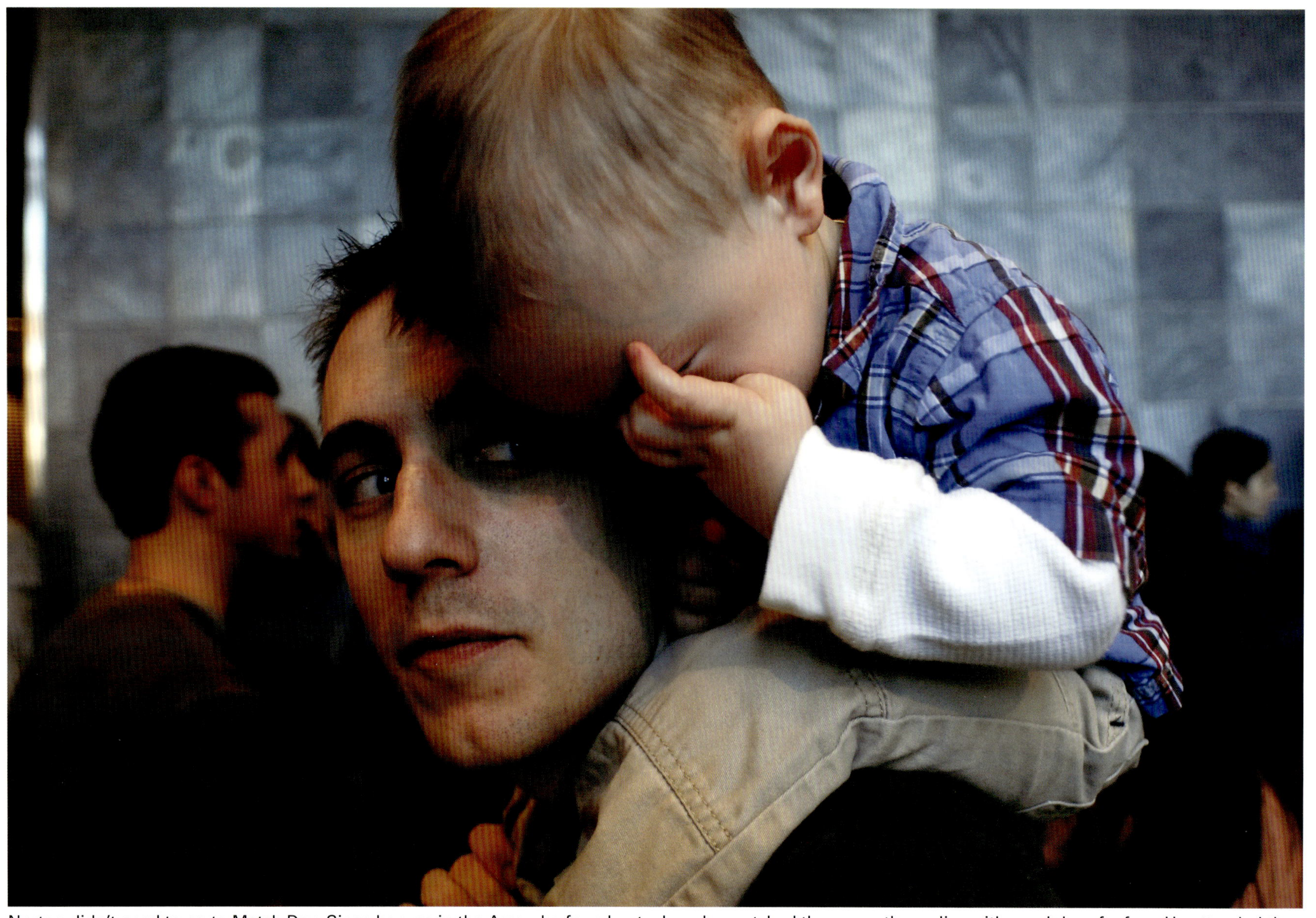

Norton didn't need to go to Match Day. Since he was in the Army, he found out where he matched three months earlier with much less fanfare. He attended the event—with son Robby—because he wanted to see where his classmates matched and celebrate with them.

match. Often, it's not because they did anything wrong; it's because an algorithm determined they weren't as good a fit as someone else. But sometimes medical students set themselves up for failure by not ranking enough programs. Between ten and twenty is the norm, more for competitive specialties, according to Dr. Charles Kent Smith, Case Med society dean and senior associate dean for students.

Gentry ranked five.

To her, even five was too many. She only wanted Maricopa Medical Center, a county hospital in Phoenix about an hour away from her parents. She wanted to see more of her mother, but she was also missing home. She had been away nearly ten years. She wanted to shop at Scottsdale Fashion Square and eat the best refried beans on the planet.

Gentry visited Maricopa in the fall. Afterward, she kept replaying the message the residency coordinator left on her voicemail. "You were very well liked," the coordinator said. "We scored you very high." She even tried to schedule another visit, known as a "second look." But it was the winter holidays, and no one called her back until January. Over the phone, the residency director asked, "Why this county hospital in central Phoenix?" She told him the truth: the program impressed her, the people were nice, and it was home.

In January, she used frequent-flier miles to get back to Maricopa. Afterward, the residents e-mailed her, telling her how much everyone liked her. Gentry had a good feeling she would be Maricopa's top-ranked candidate. She wouldn't know for sure until Match Day. At Case, Match Day is a big celebration, the kind of self-congratulatory shindig Gentry hates. She didn't think she would go, no matter what.

"It's so competitive, and these programs are so small," she worried aloud over coffee one morning, tears pooling in her eyes. "I don't know if I'll have a job."

Around noon on Black Monday, Gentry's Blackberry dinged. She shouldn't have been in bed at this hour, but insomnia had kept her up much of the night. She rolled over, picked up her phone, and clicked on the new e-mail.

"Congratulations, you have matched!"

She didn't call anyone or even jump out of bed. She just rolled back over. She was headed to Maricopa. She was so sure of it, in fact, she could finally sleep.

•◆◆◆•

Around noon on Black Monday, Franco took a lunch break during her geriatrics rotation at the Cleveland Clinic and checked her e-mail in the library. She, too, had matched. But she had no idea where. Franco had interviewed for pediatrics residencies at thirteen hospitals, including Johns Hopkins, Stanford, and Brown, her alma mater. She liked several programs, including Rainbow Babies and Children's Hospital. But one truly impressed her: Children's Hospital of Philadelphia (CHOP), ranked the best children's hospital in the nation by *U.S. News and World Report* for the past six years.

Franco considered CHOP a reach. Ever since she'd wandered the emergency department in the hospital where her mother had worked when she was a child, intrigued by the gore and fascinated by the action, she'd known medicine was the right field for her. She sought medical opportunities every chance she got. (When her beloved goldfish died, she cut it open with a butter knife just to see what was inside.) But parts of medical school had been so difficult—failing biochemistry and pulmonology in her first year, fighting depression in her third. After how far she'd come, she wasn't going to fail. For weeks, she obsessed over her Match Day results. She counted down the days on her Facebook page. The night before Match Day, she mumbled the word "Philly" in her sleep.

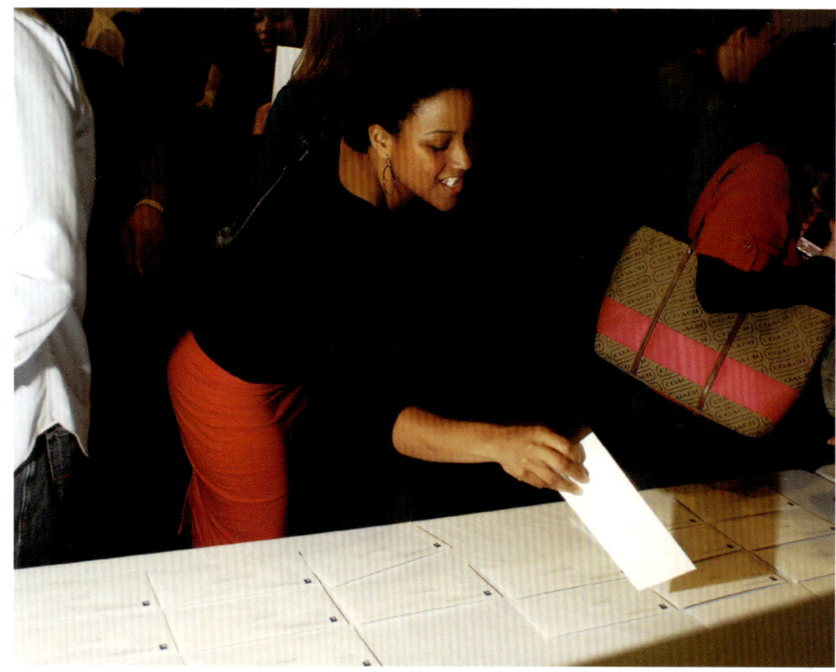

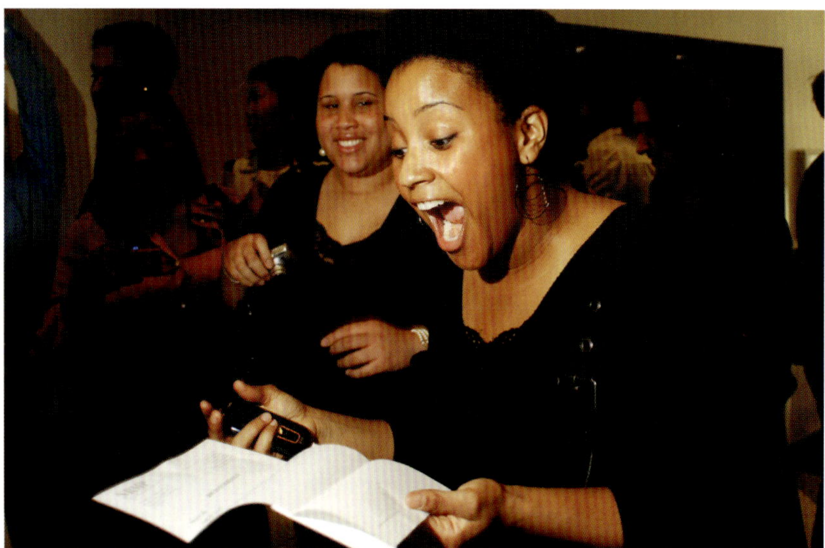

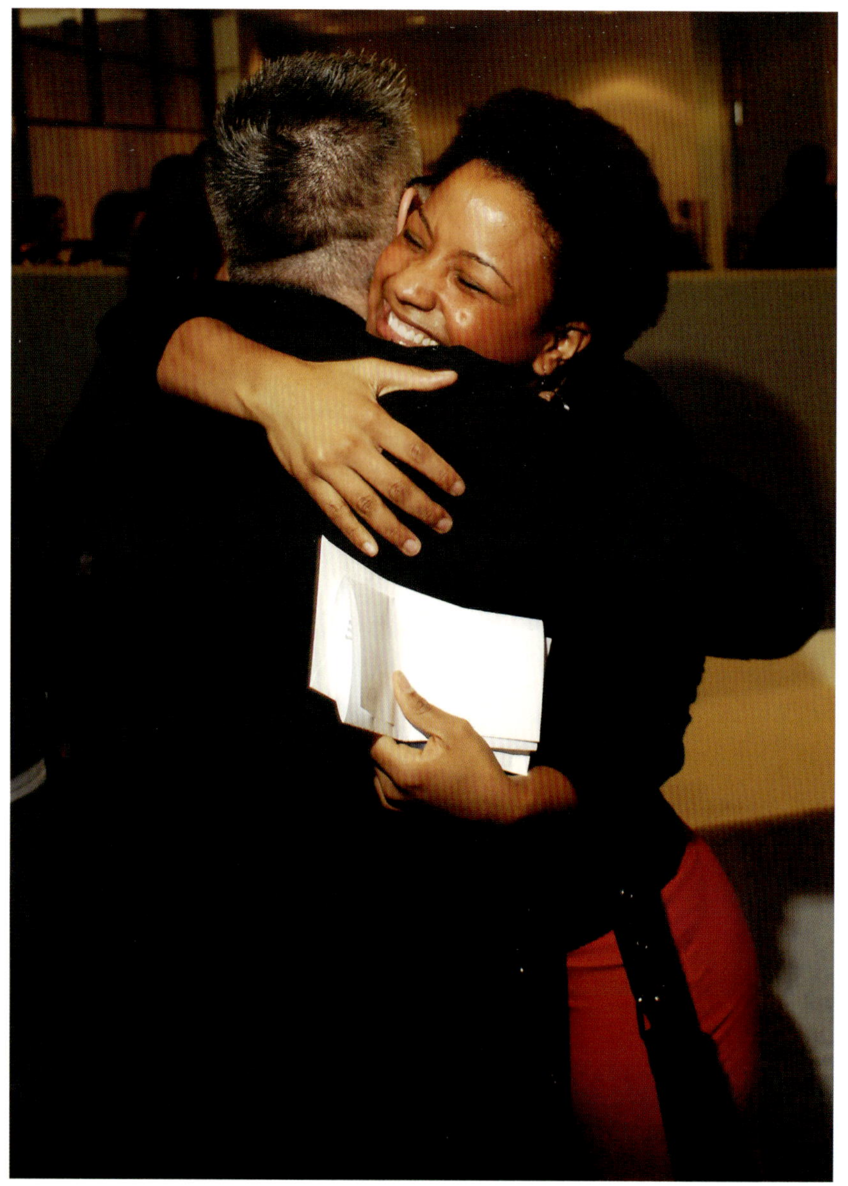

The three stages of Match Day as Franco experiences it on March 19, 2009: anticipation, surprise, jubilation.

She got up early, along with her mother and her sister, Jade, who'd come to Cleveland for this occasion. They arrived at the Iris S. & Bert L. Wolstein Research Building around 11 A.M. The envelopes waited on tables in an area sectioned off by a ribbon. Franco walked over to hers and took its picture. She couldn't decide how to open the letter: Alone in a corner where no one could see her reaction? Surrounded by her family and friends? Maybe Jade should open it.

She pulled out her cell phone and checked the time. The closer it got to noon, the tighter the students and their families squeezed into the light-drenched area where the envelopes beckoned.

Around 11:45 A.M., the first of many speakers took the microphone, trying to fill the last few minutes of an agonizing three-week-long wait. Dean Pamela B. Davis congratulated them on "an extraordinary match." She joked that trampling her during the rush for the envelopes would put them at risk of not graduating.

As another dean assured the students they would remember this day for the rest of their lives, Franco was no longer paying attention. She and a friend were strategizing the envelope opening. "We're going to get the envelope, and I think we're going to convince one another that it's OK," Franco explained.

Finally, at noon, the ribbon was cut. The crowd surged forward. Franco elbowed her way to the envelope that had her name on the outside and her future on the inside. Someone yelled, "Yes!" Someone else squealed. People cried and cheered. Jade urged her to just open it.

"God!"

"CHOP?"

"Yes!"

"I told you! I told you . . . I told you."

"Oh my God," Franco said, her voice breaking. "Congratulations. You've been matched with Children's Hospital of Philadelphia."

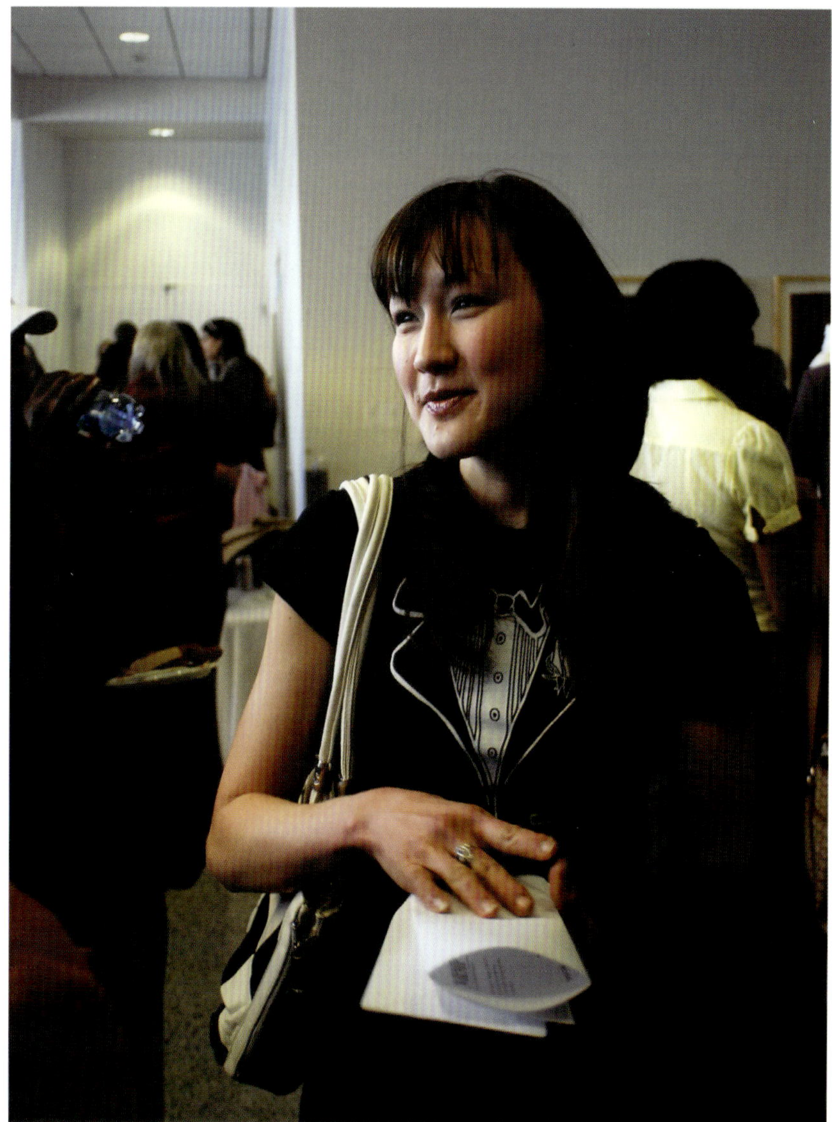

Despite all her anxiety over the match, Gentry intentionally missed the stampede to the letters, which hold the answer to the question on everyone's mind: Where did I match? Gentry knew she matched, and she felt certain she knew where. She didn't want any extra drama.

Then, the tears were hers. So were the shouts of joy, and the hugs that went on and on. One of those hugs was from assistant registrar Theresa Hancock. "No one's matched at Philadelphia in ten years," she said. "Not since I've been here. She's the first one, and that's why I'm so proud of her. She drove me crazy. Oh my God, I'm so proud of her."

Out of 175 students, the most (fifteen) matched to University Hospitals in conjunction with Louis Stokes Cleveland VA Medical Center. Seven matched to the Cleveland Clinic, and two to MetroHealth. Others matched at Duke, Yale–New Haven Hospital, Harvard Longwood, Stanford, Beth Israel Deaconess, and Johns Hopkins, among others.

At 12:20 P.M., a tall young woman in tuxedo pants, a tuxedo T-shirt, and black Chuck Taylors walked into the building alone. Gentry had decided she wanted concrete evidence of what she felt she already knew. She found her envelope quickly—there weren't many left on the table, all neatly spaced and pristine. She opened it as if she were opening the telephone bill.

It said just what she expected: Maricopa. She would start in 2010. First she would complete the first year of her residency, called a preliminary medicine internship, at St. Joseph's Hospital, also in Phoenix.

Although plenty of people remained in the building, still congratulating one another and ogling the match lists that had been taped up for public view, no one paid attention to Gentry's moment, which was just as she wanted it. There were no hugs, no cake. Just sweet relief.

The Doctors

On a pretty spring Sunday afternoon, a bright-blue procession stretched from Veale Center to Severance Hall. Bagpipes played. Children waved. Toward the back of this quickly moving line, Gentry filed past the hospitals and full parking garages of Adelbert Road. She wore battered kelly-green Chuck Taylors with a gown she'd put on for the first time that day and a cap that wouldn't stay on her head.

She talked about doing something mildly inappropriate in the $186 rental regalia. Bowling, perhaps. Or grocery shopping. It was too late for anything more involved. "Shenanigans is now professional misconduct," she quipped.

In many ways, she was the same young woman who'd arrived late to the White Coat Ceremony, the symbolic start to medical school, four years ago. The middle daughter of grocery store owners from Florence, Arizona, Gentry would still rather have two kids and a minivan than a Nobel Prize.

But on graduation day, from the ankles up, she looked like all the other graduates wearing blue gowns with velvet bands on their sleeves and fussing with their hats. They carried green hoods that, aside from matching Gentry's sneakers, identified them as new doctors of medicine.

"Holy mom," she said, not for the last time that day. "They made us doctors."

The procession of graduates met an exuberant crowd inside Severance Hall. Photographers leaned over the second-floor balcony

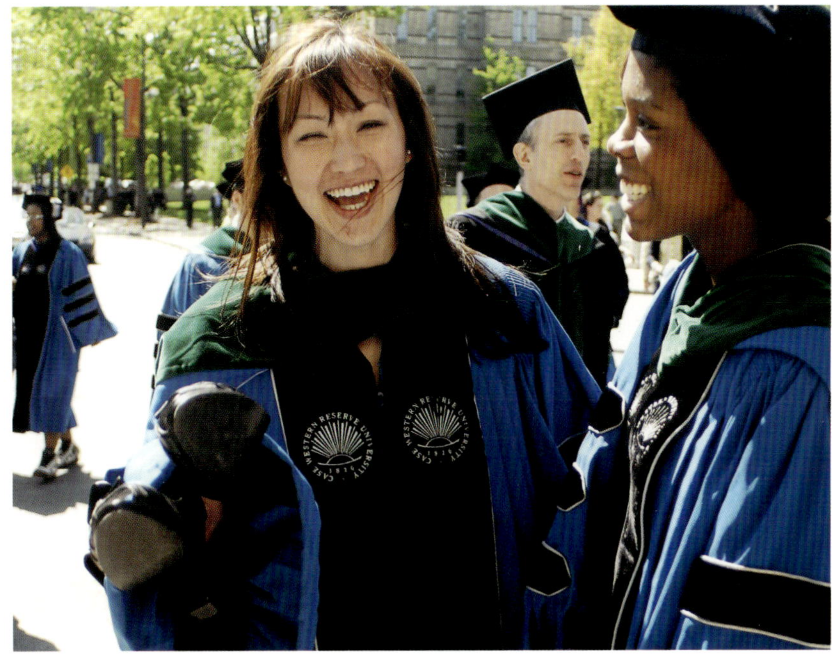

On the walk from the university-wide convocation in Veale Center to the diploma ceremony in Severance Hall, Gentry keeps saying, "Holy mom, they made us doctors!"

taking shots. Thumbs were raised high in the air. A sense of "I did it!" wafted through the crowd.

Norton walked toward the front of the line, eyes fixed toward the stage. He looked much older than he had the last time I saw him in Severance Hall. At the White Coat Ceremony, he was the guy who

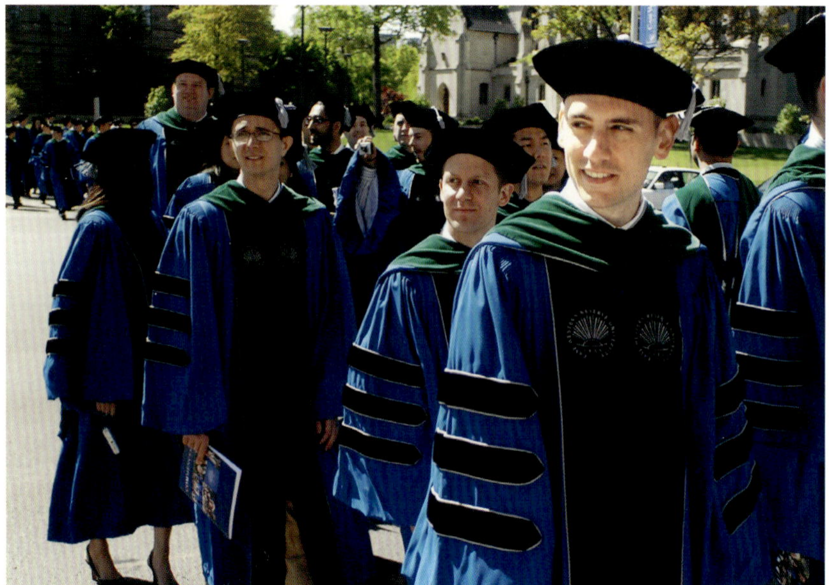

The procession moves quickly down Adelbert Road. Norton hoped his father, who was wheelchair-bound then, would find a spot in Severance Hall where he would be able to see him get his diploma.

wasn't at the party the night before; at commencement, he was a father of two. "Medical school has both demystified and elevated doctors in my view," Norton would tell me later, when I asked him how he felt on graduation day. "A doctor was always the guy you could go to who had all the answers crammed into his brain." He didn't feel that way anymore. In medical school, he'd seen attending physicians swivel in their chairs and rub their heads in frustration. He'd heard them say, "Crap, I don't know what to do. What do you think?"

To Norton, what doctors lost in deification, they gained in humanity. A doctor knows death will win sometimes, but he does everything he can to help his patient, even if it means staying later, working harder, and sacrificing more. When Norton was called to receive his diploma on the stage, his picture flashed across the screen. It included his wife, Kate; three-year-old daughter, Megan; and eighteen-month-old son, Robert Bryan II. It was taken on the porch of the Cleveland duplex they would soon leave for El Paso, Texas.

Besides the two kids, something else stood out about Norton's photo: the word "Army" in the caption. He was going to William Beaumont Army Medical Center first for one year, then to Brooke Army Medical Center in San Antonio, where he would complete his anesthesiology residency. Norton was now an active-duty Army captain, though he did not yet have the haircut. His stipend had helped the family substantially. In addition to paying for his third and fourth years of medical school, the army would compensate him $60,000 for his residency this year. In a civilian hospital, he'd earn about $10,000 to $20,000 less. If Norton chose to stay in the service longer than the three years he would owe following residency, the government would begin to take over the loans he'd incurred during his first two years of medical school, before he joined.

Norton said that since doing rotations at two Army hospitals, his biggest concerns before he joined—the war in Iraq—had lessened, even as he'd become more certain of his future deployment. "In anesthesia, if there's a conflict anywhere in the world, I'm getting deployed," he said. "They need battlefield care." He'd rather stay home, of course. But so would everyone. "At the military hospitals, I saw lots of doctors who had been deployed," he said. "All of them said they were glad they could serve the soldiers."

Though it was nothing like what he'd encounter in battle, Norton had already experienced his share of trauma during his time at MetroHealth Medical Center.

On his last day in the emergency department during his last year in medical school, he'd seen a ten-month-old whose brother had

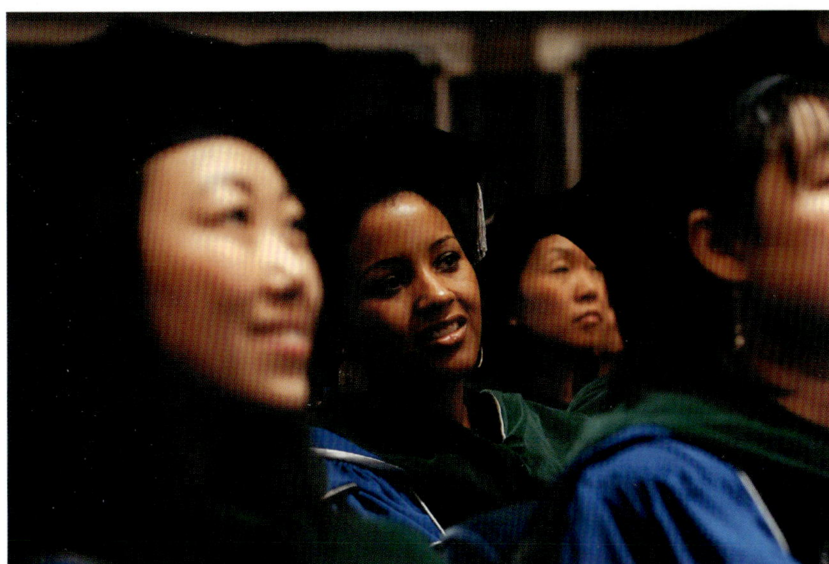

Getting hooded is the highlight of the graduation ceremony. Franco arranged for her longtime mentor, Bob Klein, to hood her, even though it's not typical for a physician who's not a faculty member or a close relative to bestow the honor.

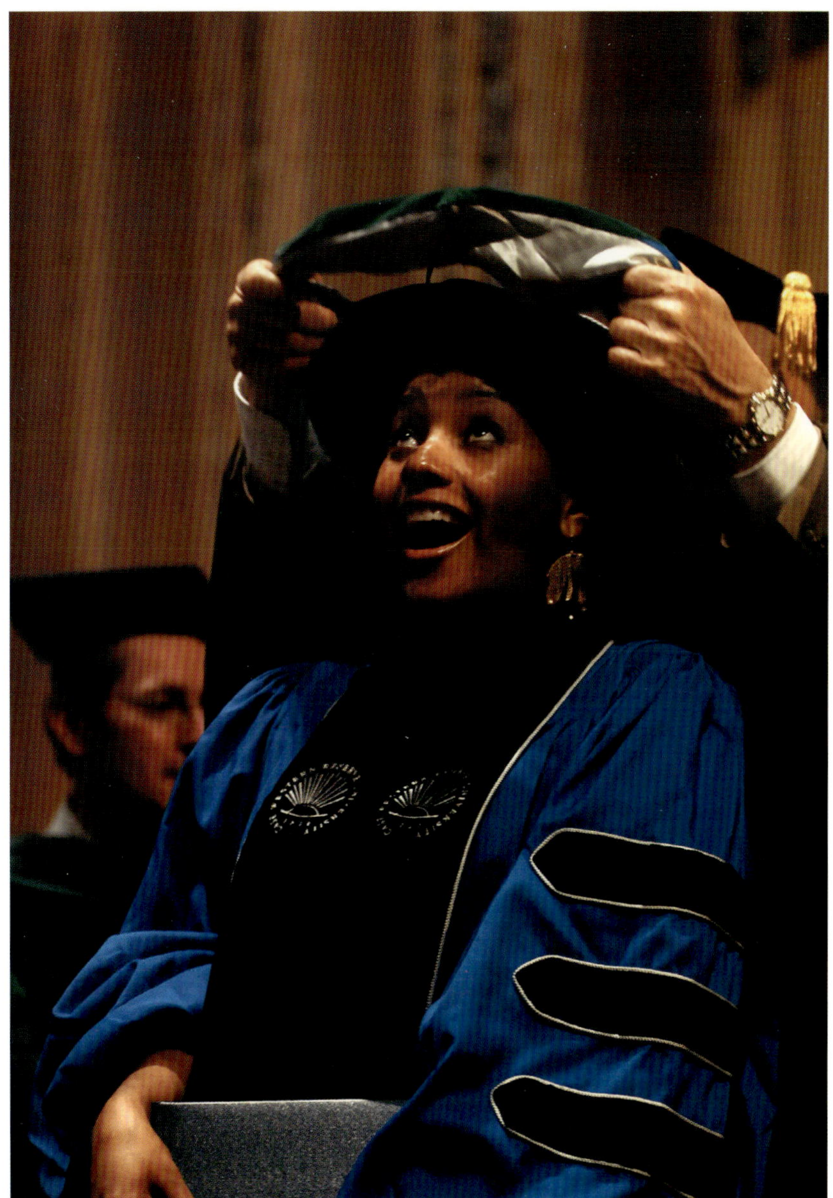

sprayed Shout in her eyes and an overweight man in his twenties with chronic headaches and chest pain. He had stapled shut a head wound and completed an arterial blood draw in one poke. Around 7:40 P.M., an ambulance brought in a forty-eight-year-old woman who had stopped breathing, her eyes glassy, her blood pressure 40 over 30. A paramedic squeezed a bag connected to the tube down her throat, getting the air into her lungs. Another walked alongside the stretcher, doing chest compressions.

The emergency team gave her epinephrine to stimulate her heart. Someone placed the sticky pads on her chest.

"Clear!"

The patient's body jumped just a little, not like in the movies. Her heart started beating, weakly, then stopped. They did CPR. They tried more drugs. They did CPR again. Norton helped find her pulse so they could get an arterial line in. Like the children's game of Pin the Tail on the Donkey, it took several tries before they finally got a line in her femoral artery.

When the patient's heart stopped for the last time, they pulled the sheet up to her neck. They closed her eyes and cleaned the vomit off her face. In the trauma bay window's reflection, Norton could see the patient's son, a man about his age, sobbing with his father.

Death is an ugly thing to behold. In his doctor fantasies, he was always beating it back. Death wouldn't win unless he lost hope. This was what he'd learned from watching his father fight ALS. Norton's parents still lived in Oregon. Every time he saw his father, he noticed another function lost. At first, he just couldn't run anymore. Then he couldn't walk. Sometimes he needed Norton's mother to translate. (Before long, he would have to get a special computer that talked for him, then a brace to put on his finger so he could hold a pencil he needed to reach the button to make it talk.) Mentally, his father was still sharp. He didn't want anyone to fuss over him. His father was an optimist. Norton, on the other hand, had never been a hope-for-the-best kind of guy. He needed to know what was going to happen and work as hard as possible to secure a good outcome. That was why he obsessed over studying for the boards, even though he did well in all the subjects they covered. On graduation day, he was applying this work ethic to hope, working at keeping it despite what he knew about this disease that would kill his father.

At the diploma ceremony in Severance Hall, Dean Davis asked the graduates to turn around and salute their families. Norton didn't expect to see his father, who should have been sitting at the back of the balcony, where there was wheelchair access. But his father had managed, somehow, to get to the front.

Norton immediately found his father's eyes and, for a moment, they lifted him up.

•◆◆◆•

In my last article on the medical students for *Cleveland Magazine,* I called Gentry a "rebel in sneakers." Her fashion statement—sneakers with formal regalia—reflected her stubborn defense of her individuality, which she felt was constantly threatened in med school. Yet, as I was writing this book, I realized I could have called all three students rebels (even though the other two students wore traditional footwear to the ceremony). Franco rose above societal barriers—economic, ethnic, and cultural—to take her place among the class of 2009. On a smaller scale, Franco bucked a tradition by having her longtime mentor Bob Klein place the hood around her neck, typically an honor afforded only to faculty members and close relatives who are physicians. Norton too fought for the MD. First, his condition, ADHD, had to be reckoned with, followed by his father's ALS diagnosis. He was becoming a doctor because he wanted to heal people; at the same time, he was coming to terms with his father's impending death, something no doctor could stop.

I came across more rebellion in the medical education literature, especially the recent reports from the Carnegie Foundation and the Macy Foundation. Some of the most respected names in medical education were calling for change, citing very compelling evidence and aiming the spotlight not just on educators but on hospital administrators, professional organizations, and policy makers.

As I read the Carnegie report, I kept thinking about my first meeting with former Case Med School dean Ralph Horwitz in 2005 and how forward thinking his approach to curriculum reform was at the time. He told me then that Case was moving away from the lecture-

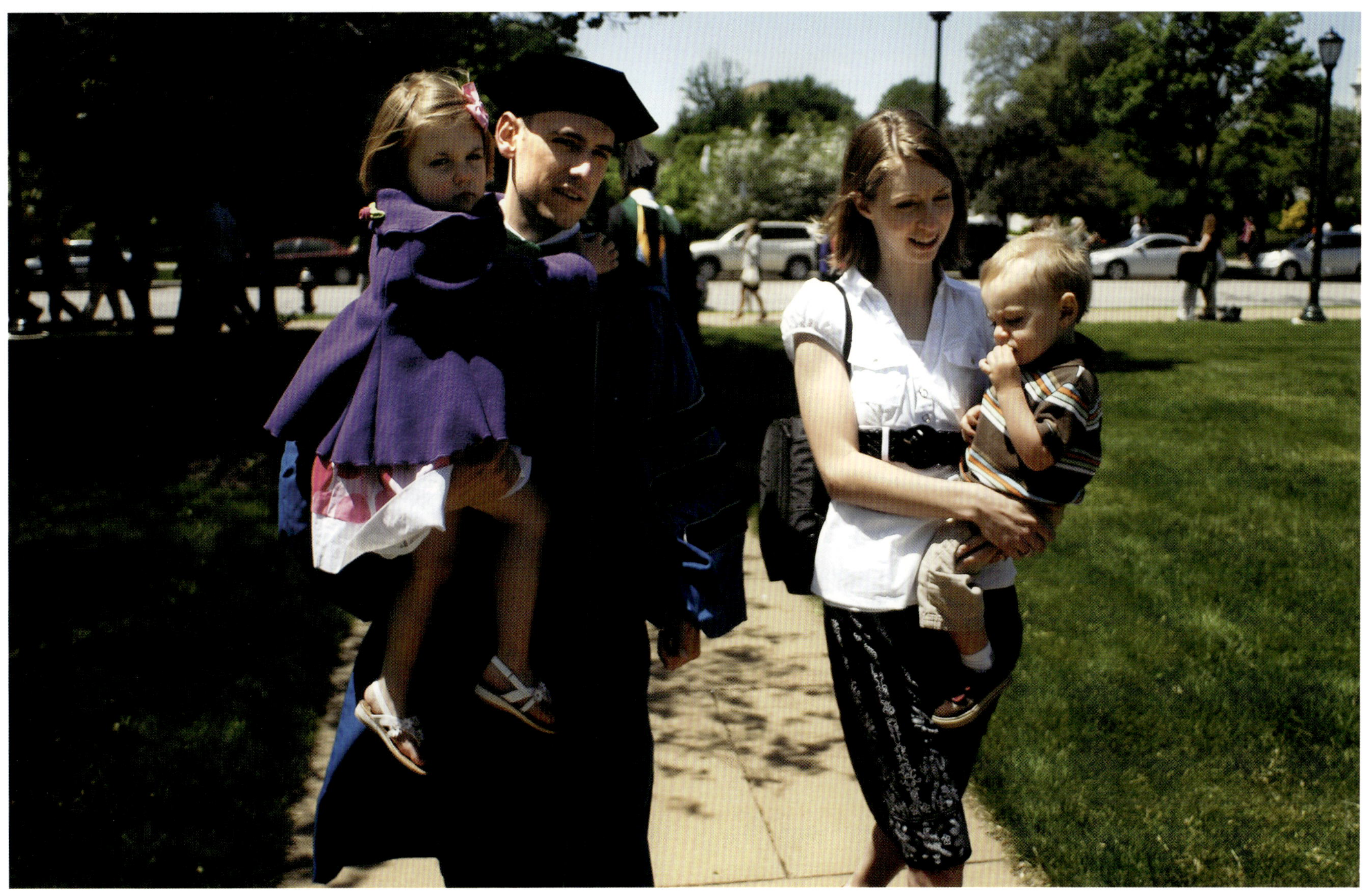

Norton and Kate carry Megan, three, and Robby, two, to the outdoor gathering at which families reunite with their new graduates.

based learning model toward one that was more collaborative. He stressed the importance of research, professionalism, and continued self-directed learning. Five years later, the 2010 report by the Carnegie Foundation for the Advancement of Teaching, which is sometimes called "Flexner II," ended up underscoring the importance of many changes Case had already instituted: the standardization of learning outcomes over learning experiences, the focus on self-directed learning, more clinical experience, and greater attention to the development of professional values. When Case administrators read the report, they chuckled. "We were way ahead of them," said Dr. Pamela B. Davis, the current dean. "We started worrying about this around the turn of the century," she said. "The notion was, the world has changed, electronic access is becoming more prevalent, the huge explosion of information. How do we prepare our students, not for today, but for twenty years from now? . . . We have to give Ralph [Horwitz] an enormous amount of credit for pushing us on and rolling the curriculum out when many people didn't think it was ready. You know, 'Not ready for primetime.' Well, you know what, if you wait until you're ready, you'll never be ready."

While this stamp of approval means a lot to the school, it's still too early to tell if and how its new graduates will change medicine. When Drs. Michael Norton, Marleny Franco, and Millicent Gentry left medical school in 2009, they entered a health-care system on the brink of change. The president had pledged reform by the end of his first year in office, and how doctors would be affected remained unclear. No matter what happens with reform, it won't lessen the expectations of people who wear the long white coats: they must save lives, or at least improve them. This perception exists despite the grim reality of American health care today. "Americans generally recognize now that our nation's health care system has become excessively expensive, ineffective, and unjust," wrote T. R. Reid, author of the 2009 *New York Times* best seller *The Healing of America: A Global Quest for Better, Cheaper, and Fairer Health Care.* "Among the world's developed nations, the United States stands at or near the bottom in most important rankings of access to and quality of medical care." Fewer deaths were prevented with timely and effective care in the United States than in eighteen other industrialized nations. Access to health care here has declined since 2006.

This wasn't all doctors' fault, though medical educators tell students they must change things. The members of the class of 2009, pioneers of the new curriculum that integrated the studies of medicine and public health, are supposed to be the new community-minded doctors the twenty-first century needs. They learned that no one grows into the white coat in four years. The coat itself needs to stretch—and keep stretching—to fit in all the new knowledge and need, all the expectations and change.

New doctors need to wear the coat the best they can.

Franco planned to wear it with an afro. The 'fro wasn't a fashion statement; it was a sign she'd overcome the language and culture barriers that keep so many people from achieving their dreams.

Norton would wear his coat in the military as he treated patients suffering from some of the worst injuries imaginable. He would wear it with hope, in his father's memory.

Gentry planned to wear her coat with sneakers. They were proof that you can get a medical degree *and* have a life. They symbolized victory over the conformists, including the doctor who said that wearing Chuck Taylors, even brand-new ones, to clinic was inappropriate. They were victory over the gunners, the students who

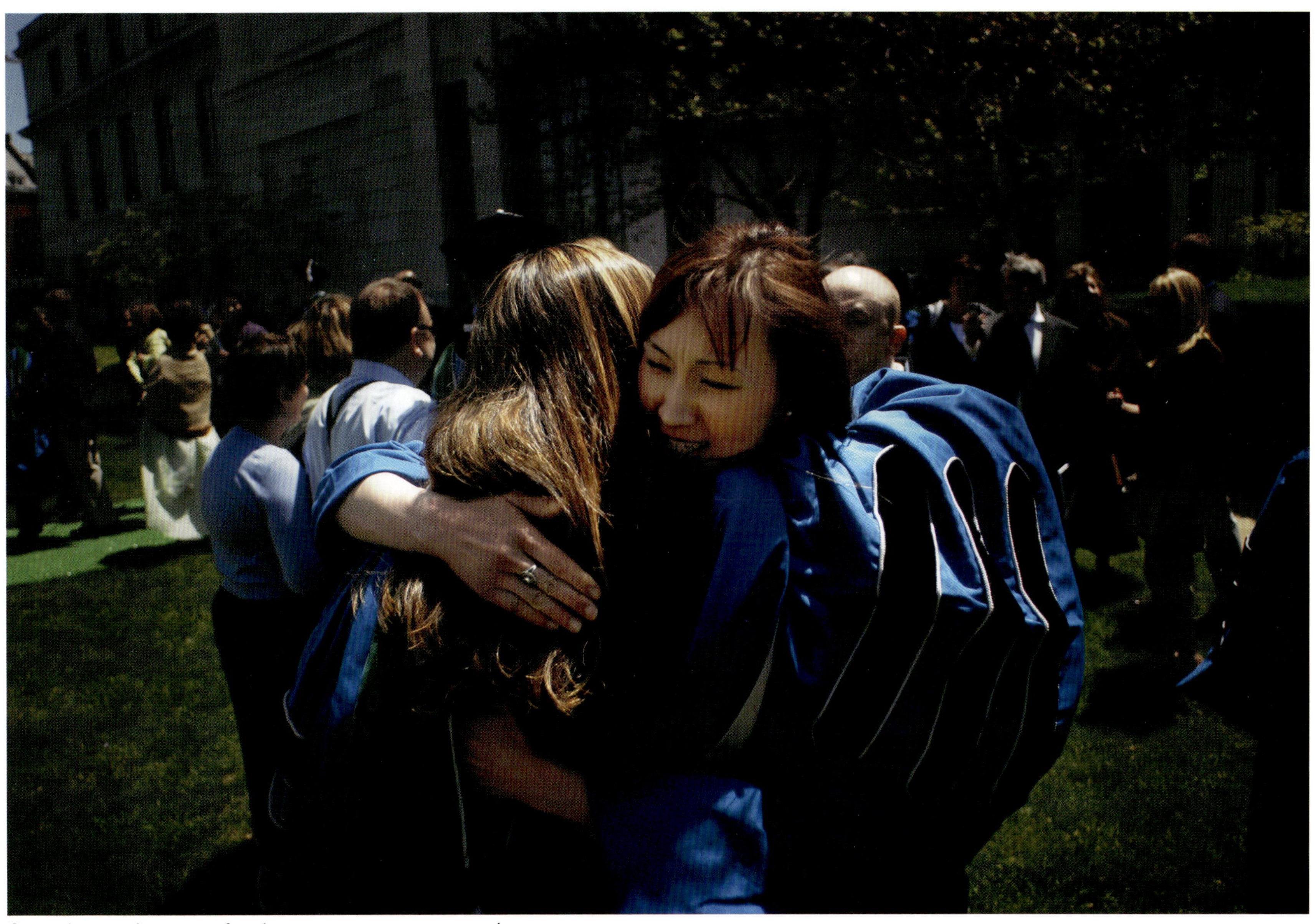

Gentry hugs a classmate after the commencement ceremonies.

excelled at medicine at the expense of their social lives and overall humanity. The sneakers were even victory over the voice she couldn't quiet at night, the one saying, *What if I fail?*

While preparing for perhaps the most difficult medical school year of all—the internship—Gentry planned to enter her tequila-crusted jalapeno-apple pie in the county fair. When it came to pie, she was a gunner. Medicine was work. Baking was living. "I'd rather be successful at life and experience life than be the world's most decorated physician," she said.

At medical school's end, Gentry had realized she'd wasted a lot of time being miserable. As with many diagnoses, if she had confronted her problem earlier, she would have had a better time of it. Attitude affects experience. She'd seen that in patients. Why didn't she see it in herself? If she had fought less and learned more in medical school, she could have had an easier time. We're not talking surrender here, more like active collaboration—finding a way to work together instead of against one another. This kind of collaboration is exactly what doctors, educators, professional organizations, hospital administrators, and even policy makers must do in order to put medical education in sync with the needs of society.

Before Gentry made her final medical school journey, the trip to the stage to get her diploma, she took off her sneakers.

She pulled four-inch heels from a bag under her gown and slipped them on.

Epilogue

Mike Norton's father died on August 28, 2009, four months after Norton received his doctorate of medicine. Robert Bryan Norton was posthumously made an honorary member of the David Satcher Society, the first honorary member of a Case academic society. Norton will complete his anesthesiology residency at Brooke Army Medical Center in San Antonio in June 2013. The Nortons are now a family of five. Daughter Elise Rachel was born on June 7, 2011.

Marleny Franco's pediatrics residency at Children's Hospital of Philadelphia concludes in 2012. She plans to do a fellowship in pediatric emergency medicine. After that, she hopes to pursue a career in academic medicine because she wants to combine a pediatric emergency practice with teaching. She says she loves many things about being a doctor, especially developing relationships with her patients and their families.

Millie Gentry is still trying to find a workable balance between her career and her personal life, which now includes a cat and a boyfriend. She will finish her radiology residency at Maricopa Medical Center in 2014 and plans to do a fellowship in women's imaging. She has not won any pie contests lately, but she's still baking. At work, she knows everyone's birthday and tries to bring cupcakes for each one.

While changes continue to be made at the Case Western Reserve University School of Medicine, Dean Davis said the school remains focused on teaching students "how to think like a doctor." That means more interprofessional learning, such as a grant-funded program in which students from the medical school and the nursing school are collaborating at the Free Medical Clinic of Greater Cleveland. She also supports an "urban health track," where every student makes a house call.

The demand for a Case medical education remains high. In 2012, there were 5,293 applicants for 196 short white coats.

Acknowledgments

I have many people to thank for their help with this project. The deans of the Case Western Reserve University School of Medicine let me and photojournalist Tim Harrison into every learning setting at the school. George Stamatis fielded my initial request and helped me secure the access we needed. Drs. Dan Wolpaw, Terry Wolpaw, and Robert Haynie spent hours with me explaining curricular changes at the school. I am inspired by their devotion to improving medical education.

Since a huge part of medical training takes place in hospitals and community-based clinics throughout the community, this story could not have been reported if not for the willingness of the doctors, nurses, and communications staff at University Hospitals, the Cleveland Clinic, MetroHealth Medical Center, and the Veterans Administration Hospital. They welcomed me into their facilities and handled the awkward conversations—and the paperwork—with patients, who had to approve of my observing their health-care treatment experiences.

I thank curator James M. Edmonson and archivist Jennifer Nieves at the Dittrick Medical History Center for leading me to some fascinating medical history. Helen Conger and Jill Tatem at the University Archives helped me put medical education at Case into historical context.

Of course, Tim and I are most indebted to Marleny Franco, Mike Norton, and Millie Gentry for allowing us into their lives at a very challenging time and never telling us to go away. They even acted as intermediaries with hospitals, professors, and patients. I owe a special thanks to some of the students' family members, including Mike's wife, Kate.

On a personal level, I must thank the people who reviewed early drafts and made the final work so much better: *Cleveland Magazine* editor Steve Gleydura for all his guidance on the magazine series, as well as two other editors at the magazine, Erick Trickey and Jim Vickers, who spent countless hours reviewing manuscripts and making suggestions to better the work. I am forever indebted to Stuart Warner, Anne Trubek, and Bob Batchelor for reading and commenting on drafts of the book. The detail-oriented and irreplaceable Justin McCraw, my former graduate assistant, helped with research and kept me on track with my classes while I finished the manuscript in 2010.

My mother and father, Lucy and Jack Marino, as well as my sister, Elizabeth, offered support in the form of babysitting, food, and constant encouragement. My mother-in-law, Dorothy Naymik, rushed to the library to read each *Cleveland Magazine* installment. She reminded me almost every time I saw her of the importance of my subject matter (and also did some babysitting).

I couldn't have produced this work without the support of my husband, Mark Naymik, with whom I share my wonderful life and passion for storytelling. Many kisses and hugs to our daughters, Stella and Charlotte, who have never known me when I wasn't working on this project. They love their doctors—and doctors in general—and I hope that never changes.

Notes

Prologue

xi Doctors used to wear black: Mark S. Hochberg, "The Doctor's White Coat—An Historical Perspective," *Virtual Mentor* 9, no. 4 (April 2007): 310.

xi At that time, getting a medical education was not difficult: Kenneth M. Ludmerer, *Time to Heal: American Medical Education from the Turn of the Century to the Era of Managed Care* (New York: Oxford University Press, 1999), 4; Hochberg.

xi In Ohio, preceptors did not require human dissection: Frederick Clayton Waite, *Western Reserve University Centennial History of the School of Medicine* (Cleveland, Ohio: Western Reserve University Press, 1946), 113.

xi "The most intimate of America's great symphony halls": Charles Michener, "The Clevelanders," *New Yorker,* Feb. 7, 2007, 44.

The Student

3 Medical students are more prone to depression: Julie M. Rosenthal and Susan Okie, "White Coat, Mood Indigo—Depression in Medical School," *New England Journal of Medicine* 353 (Sept. 15, 2005): 1085–88.

3 Narrative journalist Anne Hull has described the ethical dilemmas: Anne Hull, "A Dilemma of Immersive Journalism," in *Telling True Stories: A Nonfiction Writers' Guide from the Nieman Foundation at Harvard University,* ed. Mark Kramer and Wendy Call (New York: Penguin, 2007), 182–83.

3 The current model of American medical education was established: Molly Cooke, David M. Irby, and Bridget C. O'Brien, *Educating Physicians: A Call for Reform of Medical School and Residency* (San Francisco: Jossey-Bass, 2010), 13.

3 "Even when my colleagues from work have disagreed": Atul Gawande, *Complications: A Surgeon's Notes on an Imperfect Science* (New York: Picador, 2002), 268.

5 In terms of quality: Greer Williams, *Western Reserve's Experiment in Medical Education and Its Outcome* (New York: Oxford University Press, 1980), 19.

5 "The student inherited the departmental research": Thomas Hale Ham, "Grand Rounds in Medical Education with Medical Students Up and Down the Centuries with a Crystal Ball," speech given at the dinner of the Association of American College Physicians, May 7, 1974, Atlantic City, N.J., Case Western Reserve University archives.

5 "Because of concern over the": Thomas Hale Ham, *The Student as Colleague: Medical Education Experience at Case Western Reserve* (Ann Arbor, Mich.: University Microfilms International, 1976), 15.

7 At Case, every incoming student was appointed to one of the four societies: Lois A. Bowers, "School of Medicine Launches Advising Societies," *Medical Bulletin* (Case Western Reserve University School of Medicine) 10, no. 1 (2004): 13–14.

The Science

17 But no one can learn it all: Carmen Webb and Morris Hawkins Jr., "Mastering the First Two Years," in *Taking My Place in Medicine: A Guide for Minority Medical Students,* ed. Carmen Webb (Thousand Oaks, Calif.: Sage, 2000), 26.

18 There were 5,394 journals in MEDLINE in 2010: "Detailed Indexing Statistics: 1965–2010," U.S. National Library of Medicine, http://www.nlm.nih.gov/bsd/index_stats_comp.html; Mark Ware and Michael Mabe, *The STM Report: An Overview of Scientific and Scholarly Journal Publishing* (Oxford: International Association of Scientific, Technical and Medical Publishers, 2009), 18, http://www.stm-assoc.org/2009_10_13_MWC_STM_Report.pdf.

18 "The new and most pressing problem": Howard S. Becker, Blanche Geer, Everett C. Hughes, and Anselm Strauss, *Boys in White: Student Culture in Medical School* (Chicago: University of Chicago Press, 1961), 89.

18 There was little direction from the faculty: Becker et al., *Boys in White,* 91.

20 But she had proved: Although medical schools have been trying to achieve better racial, ethnic, and socioeconomic diversity, in the area of parental income, things seem to be getting worse. In 2008, the Association of American Medical Colleges reviewed data on parental income of those entering medical school from 1987 to 2005. It reported that the median family income the respondents reported increased from $50,000 in 1987 to $100,000 in 2006. It also found that the percentage of entering students reporting family incomes in the top quintile of U.S. household income increased from 50.8 percent in 2000 to 55.2 percent in 2005 ("Analysis in Brief," *Association of American Medical Colleges* 8, no. 1 [Jan. 2008]). Some progress, at least, has been made in the area of racial diversity. But the physician workforce still isn't as diverse as the U.S. population. For instance, in 2008, only 5.8 percent of physicians were African American while the U.S. population is estimated to be 12.8 percent African American. Tracie White, "Report Lauds Stanford, UCSF for Decades-Long Efforts to Attract Minority Students," *Inside Stanford Medicine,* http://med.stanford.edu/ism/2010/april/diversity.html.

21 Interestingly, her namesake, Millicent Fenwick, also surprised and exasperated people: Amy Schapiro, *Millicent Fenwick: Her Way* (Piscataway, N.J.: Rutgers University Press, 2003), ix.

23 Salaries for some of those specialties ranged from $250,000 to more than $600,000: Christopher J. Gearon, "Doctors in Demand," *U.S News and World Report Best Graduate Schools 2007.*

The Self

29 Dr. Alfred C. Kinsey founded: "Chronology of Events and Landmark Publications," Kinsey Institute for Research in Sex, Gender, and Reproduction, http://www.kinseyinstitute.org/about/chronology.html.

31 The class of 2009 reflected the millennial generation: Sharon Jayson, "Study: Millennial Generation More Educated, Less Employed," *USA Today,* Feb. 23, 2010, http://www.usatoday.com/news/education/2010–02–24-millennials24_ST_N.htm.

32 This is called "professional identity formation": Molly Cooke, David M. Irby, and Bridget C. O'Brien, "A Summary of Educating Physicians: A Call for Reform of Medical School and Residency," Carnegie Foundation for the Advancement of Teaching, http://www.carnegiefoundation.org/elibrary/summary-educating-physicians.

The Cadaver

41 After 300 B.C., Herophilus, the father of anatomy, instituted human dissection: Theodore Vrettos, *Alexandria: City of the Western Mind* (New York: Free Press, 2001), 62.

43 In seventeenth-century America, dissection took place: O'Malley, *The History of Medical Education,* 466.

43 Massachusetts allowed medical schools: John Harley Warner and James M. Edmonson, *Dissection: Photographs of a Rite of Passage in American Medicine, 1880–1930* (New York: Blast Books, 2009), 17.

43 Because of spiking enrollment in Ohio medical colleges: Linden F. Edwards, "Body Snatching in Ohio During the Nineteenth Century," *Ohio State Archeological and Historical Quarterly* 59, no. 5 (October 1950): 333.

43 Waite estimated that corpses: Edwards, "Body Snatching," 331.

43 "Anatomy riots": Dittrick Medical History Center, Case Western Reserve University, narrative accompanying the online exhibit "Haunting Images."

43 At the latter, the father of a woman: Edwards, "Body Snatching," 329–51.

44 In 1950, Western Reserve medical students spent 280 hours: Greer Williams, *Western Reserve's Experiment in Medical Education and Its Outcome* (New York: Oxford University Press, 1980), 117.

46 "Were most often preoccupied with the possibility": Frederic W. Hafferty, *Into the Valley: Death and the Socialization of Medical Students* (New Haven, Conn.: Yale University Press, 1991), 65.

46 "Professors counseled their students to cultivate gentleness": Warner and Edmonson, *Dissection,* 9.

46 "Cadaver stories": Hafferty, *Into the Valley,* 56–57.

47 "The activities described": Hafferty, *Into the Valley,* 59.

The Preceptorship

56 In medieval Europe: Waite, *Western Reserve University Centennial History,* 4.

56 Americans who wanted a better medical education traveled to Europe for training: Ludmerer, *Time to Heal,* 4.

56 Medical education consisted of two parts: Waite, *Western Reserve University Centennial History,* 111.

56 The first medical schools in the United States existed under the auspices of colleges of arts: Waite, *Western Reserve University Centennial History,* 22.

The Boards

64 A poor correlation exists between step 1 scores and supervisor ratings during residency: Cooke et al., *Educating Physicians,* 171.

64 Attention to the "core competencies necessary for medical practice has sparked efforts": Cooke et al., *Educating Physicians,* 171.

64 "In the American colonies, there were no legal standards of proficiency": Waite, *Western Reserve University Centennial History,* 23.

64 In the 1840s in northern Ohio: Waite, *Western Reserve University Centennial History,* 8.

65 By about 1920: Cooke et al., *Educating Physicians,* 13–14.

65 The USMLE spans: Cooke et al., *Educating Physicians,* 169–71; also United States Medical Licensing Examination, *2011 Bulletin of Information* (n.p.: Federation of State Medical Boards of the United States and the NBME, 2010), 11, http://www.fsmb.org/pdf/USMLEStep3_bulletin.pdf.

65 Researchers have shown there's little evidence: Leonard S. Werner and Brian S. Bull, "The Effect of Three Commercial Coaching Courses on Step One USMLE Performance," *Medical Education* 37, no. 6 (June 2003): 527.

The Wards

70 "The life of an individual in any society is a series of passages": Arnold van Gennep, *The Rites of Passage,* trans. Monika B. Vizedom and Gabrielle L. Caffee (Chicago: University of Chicago Press, 1960), 3, 11.

72 The nation's #1 heart program: "2007 U.S. News Ranks Cleveland Clinic One of America's Best Hospitals," Cleveland Clinic, http://my.clevelandclinic.org/library/americas_best.aspx.

77 Hispanics, who are more than 14 percent less likely than whites: "Access to Health Care and Prevention Services among Hispanics and Non-Hispanics," Centers for Disease Control and Prevention," Office of Communication, Division of Media Relations, http://www.cdc.gov/od/oc/media/presskits/hhd/hlthcare.htm.

79 Medical students are most at risk of depression: Rosenthal and Okie, "White Coat, Mood Indigo."

The Match

95 In 2009, radiologists were offered an average salary of about $391,000: "2009 Review of Physician and CRNA Recruiting Incentives," Merritt Hawkins & Associates, http://www.merritthawkins.com/pdf/mha2009incentivesurvey.pdf.

95 Applicants and programs are not allowed to request one another's list: National Resident Matching Program, http://www.nrmp.org/about_nrmp/how.html.

104 I came across more rebellion in the medical education literature: Mary Hager and Sue Russell, eds., *Revisiting the Medical School Educational Mission at a Time of Expansion* (New York, Josiah Macy Foundation, 2009), http://www.macyfoundation.org/publications/publication/conference-summary-revisiting-the-medical-school-educational-mission-at-a-t.

106 Ended up underscoring the importance of many changes Case had already instituted: "Educating Physicians: A Call for Reform of Medical School and Residency," Carnegie Foundation for the Advancement of Teaching, June 2010, http://www.carnegiefoundation.org/newsroom/press-releases/educating-physicians-call-reform-medical-school-and-residency.

106 "Americans generally recognize": T. R. Reid, *The Healing of America: A Global Quest for Better, Cheaper, and Fairer Health Care* (New York: Penguin, 2009), 8–9.

106 Fewer deaths were prevented with timely and effective care: "Why Not the Best? Results from the National Scorecard on U.S. Health System Performance, 2008," Commonwealth Fund, July 2008, http://www.commonwealthfund.org/Content/Publications/Fund-Reports/2008/Jul/Why-Not-the-Best-Results-from-the-National-Scorecard-on-U-S-Health-System-Performance-2008.aspx.